THE DEATH GAP

THE DEATH GAP

HOW INEQUALITY KILLS

DAVID A. ANSELL, MD

The University of Chicago Press   CHICAGO AND LONDON

To the memory of Steve Whitman

The University of Chicago Press, Chicago 60637
The University of Chicago Press, Ltd., London
© 2017 by David A. Ansell
All rights reserved. No part of this book may be used or reproduced in any
manner whatsoever without written permission, except in the case of brief
quotations in critical articles and reviews. For more information, contact
the University of Chicago Press, 1427 E. 60th St., Chicago, IL 60637.
Published 2017
Paperback edition 2019
Printed in the United States of America

28 27 26 25 24 23 22 21 20 19   1 2 3 4 5

ISBN-13: 978-0-226-42815-4 (cloth)
ISBN-13: 978-0-226-64166-9 (paper)
ISBN-13: 978-0-226-42829-1 (e-book)
DOI: https://doi.org/10.7208/chicago/9780226428291.001.0001

Library of Congress Cataloging-in-Publication Data
Names: Ansell, David A., author.
Title: The death gap : how inequality kills / David A. Ansell, MD.
Description: Chicago ; London : The University of Chicago Press, 2017. |
Includes index.
Identifiers: LCCN 2016055405 | ISBN 9780226428154 (cloth : alk. paper) |
ISBN 9780226428291 (e-book)
Subjects: LCSH: Social medicine—United States. | Equality—Health
aspects—United States. | Poverty—Health aspects—United States. |
Racism—Health aspects—United States. | Health–Social aspects—United
States. | Health and race—United States. | Discrimination in medical care—
United States. | Medical policy—United States.
Classification: LCC RA418.3.U6 A57 2017 | DDC 362.10973—dc23
LC record available at https://lccn.loc.gov/2016055405

♾ This paper meets the requirements of ANSI/NISO Z39.48-1992
(Permanence of Paper).

CONTENTS

Part 4: The Cure

ONE STREET, TWO WORLDS

History will have to record that the greatest tragedy of this period of social transition was not the strident clamor of the bad people, but the appalling silence of the good people. Injustice anywhere is a threat to justice everywhere. We are caught in an inescapable network of mutuality, tied in a single garment of destiny. Whatever affects one directly, affects all indirectly. He who passively accepts evil is as much involved in it as he who helps to perpetrate it. He who accepts evil without protesting against it is really cooperating with it.[1]

MARTIN LUTHER KING JR.

We all die. But tens of thousands of Americans die too early. These early deaths are not random events. These deaths strike particular individuals who live in particular American neighborhoods. And while we know that people die of cancer, heart disease, and so on, this killer isn't one that we can treat with drugs, therapy, or surgery. This killer is inequality.

This is a book about inequality and its impact on longevity. Inequality triggers so many causes of premature death that we need to treat inequality as a disease and eradicate it, just as we would seek to halt any epidemic. This is bigger than a war on cancer. It requires reassessing who we are as a country and as a people. It requires that we take action against a host of offenses that rob people of their dignity and their lives.

This sounds amorphous and abstract. But it is very concrete and specific. Inequality is all around us, as are the deaths it causes. We witness it along one Chicago street.

Ogden Avenue, Chicago: A Microcosm of American Health Inequity

Ogden Avenue cuts a diagonal swath across the crisscross monotony of Chicago's street grid. This major thoroughfare began as a Potawatomi trading path that tracked from Lake Michigan through nine miles of mud, muck, and prairie to the Des Plaines River banks in the present-day town of Riverside. The Des Plaines pours into the Illinois River, which in turn flows into the Mississippi and on down to New Orleans and the Gulf of Mexico. White settlers planked the path over in the early 1800s as a defense against persistent, gluelike mud, and the City of Chicago paved it in the early 1900s. Ogden Avenue later became a critical Midwest link in the famous Route 66, a highway that connected the East and West Coasts in the early twentieth century.[2]

Although Ogden Avenue's glory days have faded, the neighborhoods it traverses offer a lens onto the impact of inequality. Ogden's four-lane asphalt, peppered with potholes, slices through an incredible diversity of neighborhoods, connecting wide-lawned western suburbs to the edge of the steel- and glass-towered Gold Coast and to some of the lowest-income, most economically distressed communities in the country. The marginalized residents of these communities don't just have different life*styles*, they have different *lives*: most critically, people who live in those western suburbs and on the Gold Coast live significantly longer than the people in the struggling neighborhoods in between. A twenty-minute commute exposes a near twenty-year life expectancy gap.[3]

In my three-plus decades as a doctor who practiced along Ogden Avenue, I learned a simple truth. Where you live dictates when you die. This is not just true in Chicago. Every region in the United States has a street or highway like Ogden Avenue. Travel Third Avenue in New York thirty blocks from the Upper East Side to Harlem, and lose ten years of life.[4] Take a short cruise along the 405 in Los Angeles, and sixteen years of life expectancy vanish.[5]

A drive along Ogden Avenue gives us a curbside view of high-mortality neighborhoods. Before gentrification transformed it, one of those struggling communities off Ogden was called Skid Row. Block upon block of dollar-a-night transient hotels and converted warehouses housed single men and women within sight of the downtown steel and glass skyscrapers.[6] These flophouses sported glamorous names—The Viceroy, Workingmen's Palace, The Gem—but accommodated mainly alcoholics, junkies, prostitutes, and the mentally ill. In 1980, during my training as a doctor, a health worker and I made a house call to one of those hotels, in search of a patient with tuberculosis who had missed an appointment. We carried the lifesaving antibiotics to dispense, if only we could find him. We scaled an unlit stairway that reeked of stale urine up to a dormitory consisting of wall-to-wall stalls, each six by four feet and crowned with chicken wire, dubbed "birdcages." Only the faintest light filtered through dirt-speckled plate-glass windows. We opened the unlocked door to our patient's birdcage and found only a metal army cot with a shabby mattress and a weathered wooden dresser. There was barely room to stand. Tuberculosis had killed the prior three occupants of this particular birdcage, and no wonder. It was a perfect environment for the disease to thrive—dark, damp, and suffocating—yet steps from the wealth of the Gold Coast. Skid Row was an epicenter for the tuberculosis and AIDS epidemics that ravaged the city in the 1980s, and the neighborhood mortality rate reflected this.[7] In the 1990s, developers razed these flophouses to erect new apartments and loft buildings catering to young professionals and aging baby boomers moving in from the suburbs.

Southwest on Ogden from the former Skid Row neighborhood is the vast West Side ghetto. It is no different from many other inner-city neighborhoods in America, with empty lots interspersed with graffiti-marked, boarded-up businesses, the blinking red neon arrows of liquor marts, iron-barred currency exchanges, catfish joints, and storefront churches on crumbling sidewalks. There are no signs of that ancient prairie trail here except the occasional black-eyed Susan that emerges in the late summer through sidewalk cracks. The mortality rate here is among the worst in the city, and the nation.

Just before Ogden enters the run-down neighborhoods of Chicago's West Side, it passes, in quick succession, the three hospitals where I have practiced internal medicine since I arrived in the Windy City in 1978: a public safety-net hospital, John H. Stroger Jr. Hospital of Cook County; a private safety-net hospital, Mount Sinai Hospital; and an academic hospital, Rush University Medical Center, my current home. My work as a doctor in these three Chicago hospitals has given me a unique vantage point on inequality and its connection to life and death. As you head southwest on Ogden, Rush appears on the east, a shiny white butterfly-shaped tower that seems to hover fourteen stories above the street and is connected by bridges to an array of hospital and research buildings that splay westward. Despite its otherworldly look, Rush was the first medical school in Chicago, chartered in 1837, two days before the city itself was incorporated.[8] Next you see, kitty-corner to the western edge of Rush, the old Cook County Hospital—"County," as the doctors called it—where generations of the uninsured and the down-and-out sought medical care. Old County, a squat, two-block-long, eight-story behemoth, now sits abandoned, boarded up and bedraggled. An eight-foot-high chain-link fence surrounds County's main entrance to keep homeless squatters from seeking shelter underneath its faded blue canopy. Its ailing yellow-brick-clad beaux-arts facade is adorned with three-story pairs of fluted ionic columns, multicolored terra-cotta cornices, sculpted faces of roaring lions and cherubs. Once an architectural gem, it is now covered in soot and held together by netting and stainless-steel straps.

When I was twenty-six years old, medical diploma in hand, I traded the lush green hills of Upstate New York for the asphalt and steel of Chicago to work at this legendary training ground for generations of doctors and nurses. I intended to stay for just three years, but the human drama and misery I witnessed compelled me to remain longer. I practiced there for seventeen years. In 2002, County was shuttered by hospital officials and replaced by the John H. Stroger Jr. Hospital, a chunky structure that sits right behind old County and serves the same population of the poor, the unwanted, and those with no other medical options.

Those two hospitals kitty-corner from each other expose the extremes of health care in America: a beautiful and expensive institution where the finest care is available, and another that has struggled at times

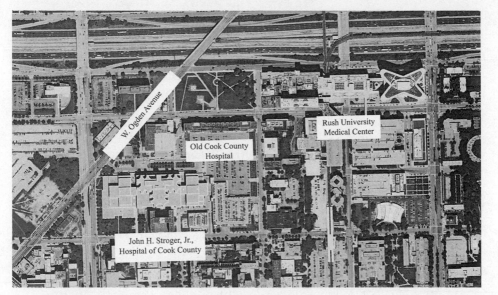

To the right of Ogden Avenue lie three hospitals: Rush University Medical Center, the shuttered old Cook County Hospital, and behind it the John H. Stroger Jr. Hospital of Cook County. Mount Sinai (not pictured) is about 0.8 mile down Ogden Avenue, on the left. Despite their close proximity to one another, large disparities exist in access to care. Source: Cook County Geographic Information Systems Center 2014.

to provide even the most basic care to poor people. My understanding of the contrasts between life and death in rich and poor patients have been deepened by my years at County and Rush. But another Ogden Avenue hospital provides a third perspective on how survival gaps have become ingrained into neighborhoods and the institutions that serve them. Continue another eight-tenths of a mile down Ogden Avenue and a railroad viaduct looms into view, spanning the roadway. Painted on it is a blue-and-white advertisement for the Sinai Health System, whose flagship institution soon appears on the left.

Mount Sinai Hospital, where I worked from 1995 to 2005, is a mismatched mass of utilitarian brick and concrete buildings that crowd the corner of Ogden and California. A Jewish industrialist established Sinai in 1919 as a hospital for the Eastern European Jews who were surging into the industrial North Lawndale ghetto.[9] During the 1950s, black migration from the Deep South transformed the community. As unscrupulous real estate agents inflamed racist fears of black people,

whites fled in droves. Lawndale flipped from an all-white neighborhood of 87,000 to an all-black one of 125,000.[10] Imagine what happens
to a community's stability when 220,000 people, the equivalent of a
medium-sized city, migrate in and out of it within a single decade.
When Dr. Martin Luther King Jr. brought his civil rights fight north
in 1966, he moved into Lawndale, just blocks from Sinai.[11] In 1968,
following King's assassination, some distraught community members torched neighborhood businesses in the anger and rebellion that
wracked the West Side for days.[12] Most of the businesses that lined
the Roosevelt Road shopping corridor near Sinai never reopened, and
within a few years the remaining industries that had provided reliable
work and health insurance to Lawndale residents fled to the suburbs.[13]
Years of disinvestment and neglect followed.

From my corner office on the ninth floor of Sinai, I could see two
brick towers that loomed over Lawndale: one to the north and one
directly west. To the north towered the Sears Roebuck Company headquarters and catalog factory, which employed tens of thousands of
people until the 1970s, when it fled to the downtown high-rise that
bore its name.[14] To the west, the decaying Hawthorne Works Tower
now lords over a working-class strip mall, with a Foot Locker, a Dol-
lar General, and an abandoned storefront clinic. The tower was once
the headquarters of a giant Western Electric plant that manufactured
electronics and phones, employing 25,000 people before it shuttered
and stripped thousands of community members of jobs and health
insurance.[15] Jobs at the mall do not have the security or the pay that the
old industrial jobs did. The flight of industry marked the beginning of
Lawndale's spiral into misery and concentrated poverty. By the 1990s,
Lawndale's population had dwindled to about 40,000. Median incomes
sank beneath the Chicago average, and the rates of uninsured grew.[16]
As a result, Lawndale's life expectancy today is among the lowest in
the Chicago region.

Lawndale is one particular neighborhood, along one particular
street, in one particular city. But the story of Lawndale is the story of
rising inequality and premature death in America's abandoned neighborhoods.

The flight of people, jobs, and wealth and the impoverishment of neighborhoods that ensued triggered America's current inequality crisis. We can trace the growth of the uninsured population and the widening death (and wealth) gaps between rich and poor, between black and white, to events like those that transpired in Lawndale. But the root of America's inequality crisis is not just the flight of people, jobs, and wealth. The active exploitation of those without resources by those controlling economic and political power in the United States subverted the ability of neighborhood residents to fight back. This fact is critical to understanding why inequality is so entwined in the tapestry of American life and so difficult to eradicate. If we are ever to reverse course, we need to understand the active nature of this exploitation. It was not just a bad economy and prejudice that crippled Lawndale and neighborhoods like it across the United States. The abusive conditions that foster inequality are perpetuated by the actions of the powerful to enrich themselves at the expense of others.[17] From the racially inflammatory blockbusting encouraged by corrupt local government and the real estate industry in the mid-twentieth century, through tax policies that have redistributed wealth from the poor and middle class to the wealthy, to the Machiavellian mass evictions, as well as the racist policing and incarceration practices of the twenty-first century,[18] the persistence of inequality in American life is not the result of random events, bad choices, or bad luck but rather the result of active acts of commission.

Hardwired Inequity

On one street, in one city, at three hospitals within one mile of one another, I discovered that inequality is hardwired into our health care delivery system and into the neighborhoods these hospitals serve. I learned from my practice along Ogden something that I was not taught in medical school: inequality itself is a cause of death. But how was I supposed to treat it? What was it about the poverty and segregation of neighborhoods like Lawndale that led to high rates of common diseases such as diabetes, hypertension, heart disease, and depression?

I was trained to treat the biological and psychological manifestations of disease, not alter the characteristics of neighborhoods. This inequality is invisible to the thousands of commuters who whiz by every day. But as a doctor, I have witnessed the suffering that inequality has inflicted on my patients and the health care institutions that serve the poor.

At Rush, the right insurance card provides access to world-class health care and just about any service imaginable. Modern biomedicine is booming at Rush as the therapeutic armamentarium grows. But if you have the wrong insurance card at Rush (or no insurance card), access to some doctors and services is blocked. At Stroger, a patient receives the best care the hospital has to offer without regard to ability to pay, but often after a mind-numbing wait. Some critical specialty services and even some basic care, such as screening mammograms and colonoscopies, are often unavailable in the county system. At Sinai, the conditions are similar to Stroger but with better access to some specialists—yet not to all. For example, both Stroger and Sinai have busy trauma units, and the mostly poor minority patients dying there donate many of the organs used in transplantation at the wealthier transplant centers across the city. Yet in my twenty-seven years at those institutions, not one of my patients—or those of my colleagues—ever *received* a lifesaving organ transplant.

At Sinai, chronic funding shortages meant that the facilities were dated and improvements always limited. While Sinai had dedicated itself to addressing the ills of the surrounding communities, it often lacked the finances to provide all the necessary care. While most financially stable not-for-profit hospitals have hundreds of days of cash reserves to support the delivery of services, during my days at Sinai we were strapped for money. The lack of cash reserves limited investment in clinical services to only the most crucial, and this inevitably affected the quality of care. Year after year, replacement of the kidney dialysis machines at Sinai was put off for lack of funds. When the federal government began to require that dialysis units report the quality of their treatments, Sinai's patients performed worse than the national average because without the right equipment, even the best doctors cannot always provide the best care. Ultimately, new machines were purchased and the quality improved.

In my seventeen years at County, not once did one of my patients who needed a joint replacement for debilitating arthritis get one. Even now, thirty years later, there is at least a five-year waiting list for joint replacements at Stroger. In ten years at Sinai, I had a number of patients with severely arthritic joints, but only two got them replaced. But at Rush, a mecca for orthopedics, you can get on the list for a joint replacement in a few weeks—provided you have the proper insurance card. The chief medical officer at the County Health System once told me, "David, the waiting list for the eye clinic at County is so long that you can go blind on it!" And yet across the street at Rush a patient can get into the eye clinic with no delay.

When I was on the front lines at County and Sinai, my patients were uninsured, black and Latino, and poor. In America that means they were often excluded from accessing the very best in treatments. I treated many patients who suffered or died early because the lifesaving treatments available just down the street were beyond their reach. I did the best I could for my patients. I rationalized that the care I was giving was good enough. But when I reached Rush and saw an institution awash in medical wealth, I knew I was wrong. It was not enough just to show up at a neighborhood clinic or a dilapidated frontline hospital if the system itself was unfair. I was the same doctor, on the same street, in the same city, and yet it was as if my patients and I had landed on another planet—one where, miraculously, they could live longer.

And as my practice took me from hospital to hospital, from clinic to clinic, I discovered that the same embedded forces that created high-mortality neighborhoods also degraded the capabilities of the health care facilities that served them. These facilities were unequal not because of the doctors or the nurses who practiced there but because of the different resources they could draw on. I found that premature illness and death are spawned in communities of immense poverty and further exacerbated by the inability of health care institutions to provide complete care as they are inundated by the uninsured. The tragic configuration of our fee-for-service system and the high rates of uninsured in the communities hardest hit by disease and death leave hospitals like County and Sinai in continual existential struggles.

One Street, Two Americas

Along that one-mile stretch of Ogden, there are two Americas of health and two Americas of health care delivery: one for those with insurance and money and another for the poor, uninsured, and dispossessed. Along this centuries-old route through Chicago's West Side, my patients and I discovered everything that was wrong with health and health care in America—not just Chicago. The health inequities seen in microcosm there extend across the United States, in every major city, in Appalachia, on Native American reservations, and in many other places. While much of this book's focus is on the urban black experience, the structural violence that undergirds health inequality is a national problem.

I came to realize this as I became a social epidemiologist. I began to study communities and social factors that lead to premature mortality and low life expectancies in Chicago. Black neighborhoods experience high degrees of hardship and have life expectancies closer to those in developing countries than those in an advanced developed nation. What had been conveniently invisible became obscenely visible as I analyzed the data. I began to ask: How could such suffering and low life expectancies coexist alongside some of the finest health care systems and some of the wealthiest neighborhoods in the nation? Was this inevitable? How have public policies, laws, and real estate practices contributed to the multigenerational poverty and high death rates in certain communities?

In many ways my insights about premature death in the neighborhoods along Ogden Avenue follow directly in the footsteps of Friedrich Engels and Rudolf Virchow, both of whom wrote in the mid-1800s about social conditions and health. Engels wrote a seminal piece on the mortality of the working class in England in which he equated the bodily injury and death that resulted from abject working conditions with manslaughter and murder. Virchow, the "father of social medicine," wrote that a typhus outbreak in the Silesia region of Prussia had

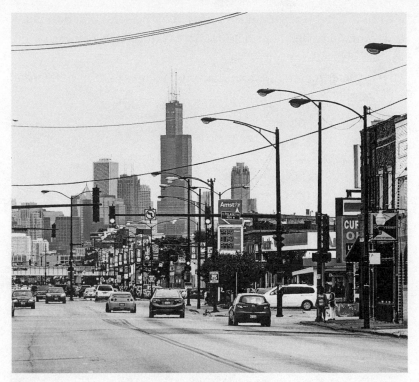

Ogden Avenue in the Lawndale neighborhood of Chicago heads east toward Chicago's Gold Coast. A Route 66 sign hangs from a lamppost just in front of the traffic signal. The life expectancy in this neighborhood is 72 years, and the average income is $25,000. The life expectancy in the vicinity of the downtown, a few miles away, is 85 years. Source: MHCooper Photography.

been caused by a lack of democracy in that region: the proper response to the epidemic was political, not medical.

This book is written in the spirit of Engels and Virchow. It is aimed at the general reading public to provide understandable explanations for the state of health and premature death in the United States, with a focus on the social and political conditions that are at the root of inequity in life expectancy. Structural violence, the corrosive combination of poverty and racism, has killed millions of Americans over multiple generations in neighborhoods of concentrated poverty. These communities have been all but abandoned while communities of concentrated wealth and advantage have thrived. This didn't have to be, and it doesn't have to stay this way. Disease and life-expectancy gaps are not inevitable or immutable. This book presents practical policy and community-building solutions that can drastically reduce or eliminate these health inequities.

With determination, we can chart a path forward to a healthier and more equitable society.

PART 1
AMERICAN ROULETTE

1

AMERICAN ROULETTE

Everyone knows that suffering exists. The question is how to define it. Given that each person's pain has a degree of reality for him or her that others can surely never approach, is widespread agreement on the subject possible? Almost all of us would agree that premature and painful illness, torture and rape constitute extreme suffering. Most would also agree that insidious assaults on dignity such as institutionalized racism and sexism also cause great and unjust injury.[1]

PAUL FARMER, MD

Windora Has a Stroke

The ear-splitting beep of my pager pierced the air. The message was from Megan, the nurse practitioner in my office: "Windora Bradley is in the office. Having a stroke. Stroke team activated. Come ASAP!"

I have been tethered to my beeper since my first day at Cook County Hospital in 1978. I still feel a jolt each time it squawks. My heart pounds. My tongue sticks to the roof of my mouth. Then a hot flush of blood rushes to my temples as an adrenaline release, triggered by the electronic pulse, bombards my nerve endings. My nervous system had long ago hot-wired my "fight or flight" reaction to the pager. It squawks, I react.

I dropped what I was doing and jogged to the stairwell that leads to my office one floor below. It had been many years since I had to run to a medical emergency. My pace was slower and less graceful now but no less determined. Windora was having a brain attack. As I skipped two-by-two down the stairs, thoughts of Windora and her illness flooded my own brain. Her tale had been a long one, though I hadn't thought it was leading us to this. Still, for the last year I had felt like a bystander at a three-alarm fire as I witnessed her body self-combust.

Windora is likely to die young because she is poor, because she is black, and because she lives in the wrong American neighborhood. She is just the latest victim of American roulette, a perverse game where the odds are stacked against the Windoras of the world.

Russian roulette is a deadly game of chance. The gambler places a bullet in the chamber of a six-shooter gun. The chamber is twirled. He places the barrel to his temple, then squeezes the trigger. His fate is determined in an instant.

American roulette is a lethal game that is played out over a lifetime in certain neighborhoods in America. How long you live depends on who you are and where you live. The early deaths that result from American roulette are not up to chance, though. The game is rigged. Live in my neighborhood—a diverse upper middle-class community just beyond Chicago's West Side—and you can on average enjoy a long and healthy life. Live on Windora's block and you will more than likely die an early death. Her medical problems were magnified by her neighborhood and life circumstances, and these are shaped as much by national forces as by local ones.

Since 1975 inequality in income, wealth, and social well-being have risen in the United States as public policies favoring the wealthy have been advanced at the expense of the poor.[2] Tax, economic, and criminal justice polices promoted by Presidents Nixon, Reagan, Bush, Clinton, and Bush II reversed rules in place since early in the twentieth century and redistributed billions of dollars from the middle class and poor to the wealthy. The War on Drugs and draconian sentencing laws led to the highest mass-incarceration rates in the history of the world. Welfare reform, Wall Street deregulation, and global trade laws passed by Congress and signed by President Bill Clinton reversed the social contract between the government and the poor in force since the Great Depression of the 1930s and the War on Poverty in the 1960s.[3] By 2005, the top 1 percent of Americans controlled more American wealth that the bottom 90 percent.[4] One family alone, the Waltons of Walmart fame, is worth $145 billion, equal to the wealth of 43 percent of American families.[5]

The American dream has disappeared for millions of Americans like Windora, who has slipped down the economic ladder over her lifetime.[6] We speak of America as a democracy, but it has become a plutocracy where members of a small minority dictate the shape of life and death in the nation through their grip on wealth. Because of their influence, the United States is vastly more unequal than other advanced industrial societies. And as inequality has increased, there has been a corresponding impact on life expectancy. Because life expectancies are so low in so many neighborhoods, the United States *as a whole* has dropped to the bottom of the world's developed countries in life expectancy.[7]

A Doctor Meets a Patient

Windora had been my patient for more than thirty years. We met in a small steaming-hot office in the General Medicine Clinic at the County Hospital. She had full cheeks, with a wide ivory-toothed smile, mahogany eyes, and silky ebony skin.

Windora and I were both twenty-seven years old then, and we had both moved to Chicago from elsewhere. But the chasm between us could not have been more stark. I was a white middle-class man from New York State. Windora had moved as a teen from Jim Crow Birmingham, Alabama, to Chicago with her parents and nine siblings. The Bradley family settled into the Cabrini Green high-rise public housing complex on Chicago's North Side and then moved to a house a few miles to the west in the Humboldt Park neighborhood. By the time Windora entered my office, her neighborhood had flipped from a mostly white and middle-class community into an all black and Puerto Rican high-poverty, high-crime one. Meanwhile, I was living in a safe, mostly white and gentrified neighborhood less than three miles away.

Still, we hit it off right away. What struck me the most, even in those early days, was her generosity and easy laugh in spite of her personal setbacks. Over time, as often happens in primary care practices, we

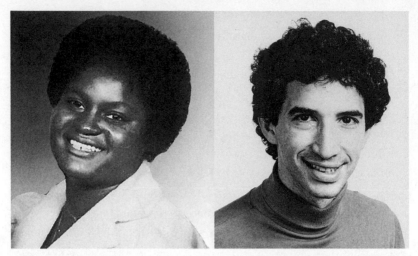

Windora Bradley and the author were both age 27 when they met. Source: author's personal collection.

became friends. We shared in each other's triumphs and tragedies. She comforted me when my father died, and I was the first person she called when her son had a cardiac arrest. Many of her family members became my patients, including four of her sisters and her son, daughter, and grandchildren. I became an unofficial member of the family.

Windora commanded a kitchen for the Chicago public school system, feeding elementary school kids, for over thirty years. Her salary was barely a living wage, yet she raised two children in her family house. When I met her, she, like so many of my patients, was obese and had just developed diabetes and hypertension. And like so many of my patients, despite working a full-time job and having insurance, she often was forced to decide between feeding and clothing her children and buying her medicine.

Tragedy and stress punctuated her entire life. Her mother and father died in their fifties from complications of diabetes. Her son died of cardiovascular disease at forty-two. Her granddaughter was murdered at the age of eight, one Easter Sunday in the alley near her house. The day before her grandnephew was to start his senior year of high school, he was shot and killed as he pushed a teenage girl out of the line of gunfire.

These events and the passage of time took a devastating toll on

Windora's body. Her blood pressure and blood sugars fluctuated wildly despite powerful medications. She developed a blockage in one of the arteries in her leg, giving her knifepoint calf cramps when she walked. Her heart raced out of control in paroxysms of chest-pounding flutters. Her skin mottled. I did what I could to manage her illnesses, but I was unable to slow the relentless course of her maladies. She was a runaway train of symptoms and disease. I was the hapless, helpless conductor.

I was trained on the biomedical model of disease, which holds that diseases arise from biological defects or imbalances in the body. Our medical and surgical therapies are directed at treating these defects. In many cases, these approaches work. Vaccinations have all but eliminated childhood diseases that once killed by the millions. Antibiotics have cured diseases that were once a scourge. Modern therapies for hypertension and atherosclerosis have seen heart-disease mortality plummet. New therapies have prolonged survival for many people with cancer. But despite these miracles of modern medicine, some American communities, like Windora's Humboldt Park, have death rates similar to those in developing countries. Why do these gaps exist?

Structural Violence

It is easy to look at Windora's brain attack through the lens of biology. Her diet, her lifestyle, and her innate biology all led to this moment when her brain is being suffocated by a blood clot in a cerebral artery. But what if it was not just biology that caused her stroke?

There are many different kinds of violence. Some are obvious: punches, attacks, gunshots, explosions. These are the kinds of interpersonal violence that we tend to hear about in the news. Other kinds of violence are intimate and emotional.

But the deadliest and most thoroughgoing kind of violence is woven into the fabric of American society. It exists when some groups have more access to goods, resources, and opportunities than other groups, including health and life itself. This violence delivers specific blows against particular bodies in particular neighborhoods. This unequal advantage and violence is built into the very rules that govern our society. In the absence of this violence, large numbers of Americans would be able to live fuller and longer lives.

This kind of violence is called structural violence, because it is embedded in the very laws, policies, and rules that govern day-to-day life.[8] It is the cumulative impact of laws and social and economic policies and practices that render some Americans less able to access resources and opportunities than others. This inequity of advantage is not a result of the individual's personal abilities but is built into the systems that govern society. Often it is a product of racism, gender, and income inequality. The diseases and premature mortality that Windora and many of my patients experienced were, in the words of Dr. Paul Farmer, "biological reflections of social fault lines."[9] As a result of these fault lines, a disproportional burden of illness, suffering, and premature mortality falls on certain neighborhoods, like Windora's. Structural violence can overwhelm an individual's ability to live a free, unfettered, healthy life.

As I ran to evaluate Windora, I knew that her stroke was caused in part by lifelong exposure to suffering, racism, and economic deprivation. Worse, the poverty of West Humboldt Park that contributed to her illness is directly and inextricably related to the massive concentration of wealth and power in other neighborhoods just miles away in Chicago's Gold Coast and suburbs. That concentration of wealth could not have occurred without laws, policies, and practices that favored some at the expense of others. Those laws, policies, and practices could not have been passed or enforced if access to political and economic power had not been concentrated in the hands of a few. Yet these political and economic structures have become so firmly entrenched (in habits, social relations, economic arrangements, institutional practices, law, and policy) that they have become part of the matrix of American society. The rules that govern day-to-day life were written to benefit a small elite at the expense of people like Windora and her family. These rules and structures are powerful destructive forces. The same structures that render life predictable, secure, comfortable, and pleasant for many destroy the lives of others like Windora through suffering, poverty, ill health, and violence. These structures are neither natural nor neutral.

The results of structural violence can be very specific. In Windora's case, stroke precursors like chronic stress, poverty, and uncontrolled hypertension run rampant in neighborhoods like hers. Windora's illness was caused by neither her cultural traits nor the failure of her will. Her stroke was caused in part by inequity. She is one of the lucky ones, though, because even while structural violence ravages her neighborhood, it also abets the concentration of expensive stroke-intervention services in certain wealthy teaching hospitals like mine.

If I can get to her in time, we can still help her.

Income Inequality and Life Inequality

Of course, Windora is not the only person struggling on account of structural violence. Countless neighborhoods nationwide are suffering from it, and people are dying needlessly young as a result. The magnitude of this excess mortality is mind-boggling. In 2009 my friend Dr. Steve Whitman asked a simple question, "How many extra black people died in Chicago each year, just because they do not have the same health outcomes as white Chicagoans?" When the *Chicago Sun-Times* got wind of his results, it ran them on the front page in bold white letters on a black background: "HEALTH CARE GAP KILLS 3200 Black Chicagoans and the Gap is Growing." The paper styled the headline to look like the declaration of war that it should have been.

In fact, we did find ourselves at war not long ago, when almost 3,000 Americans were killed. That was September 11, 2001. That tragedy propelled the country to war. Yet when it comes to the premature deaths of urban Americans, no disaster area has been declared. No federal troops have been called up. No acts of Congress have been passed. Yet this disaster is even worse: those 3,200 black people were in Chicago alone, in just one year. Nationwide each year, more than 60,000 black people die prematurely because of inequality.[10]

While blacks suffer the most from this, it is not just an issue of racism, though racism has been a unique and powerful transmitter of violence in America for over four hundred years.[11] Beyond racism, poverty and income inequality perpetuated by exploitative market capitalism are singular agents of transmission of disease and early death. As a result, there is a new and alarming pattern of declining life expectancy among white Americans as well. Deaths from drug overdoses in young white Americans ages 25 to 34 have exploded to levels not seen since the AIDS epidemic. This generation is the first since the Vietnam War era to experience higher death rates than the prior generation.[12] White Americans ages 45 to 54 have experienced skyrocketing premature death rates as well, something not seen in any other developed nation.[13] White men in some Appalachian towns live on average twenty years less than white men a half-day's drive away in the suburbs of Washington, DC. Men in McDowell County, West Virginia, can look forward to a life expectancy only slightly better than that of Haitians.[14]

But those statistics reflect averages, and every death from structural violence is a person. When these illnesses and deaths are occurring one at a time in neighborhoods that society has decided not to care about—neighborhoods populated by poor, black, or brown people—they seem easy to overlook, especially if you are among the fortunate few who are doing incredibly well. The tide of prosperity in America has lifted some boats while others have swamped. Paul Farmer, the physician-anthropologist who founded Partners in Health, an international human rights agency, reflects on the juxtaposition of "unprecedented bounty and untold penury": "It stands to reason that as beneficiaries of growing inequality, we do not like to be reminded of misery of squalor and failure. Our popular culture provides us with no shortage of anesthesia."[15]

That people suffer and die prematurely because of inequality is wrong. It is wrong from an ethical perspective. It is wrong from a fairness perspective. And it is wrong because we have the means to fix it.

Windora's Last Words

I pushed the swinging glass door to my office and hurried into the examination room to find Windora planted on a chair next to Megan. She gaped at me with a dazed, glassy-eyed stare. Sweat beaded and dripped in rivulets down her wrinkled brow.

"Windora, what's wrong?" I asked.

"Ga, ga, ga," she gargled. Something terrible was happening.

"Check her sugar," I said to an assistant. Windora was a diabetic, and low blood sugar might cause something like this.

"Who dropped you off at the hospital?"

She struggled to find her words. "Da, Da, Da, Dr. Ansell," she stuttered.

"Do you mean Darrell?" I asked. Darrell was her longtime companion. She stared at me blankly. There was fear in her gaze.

The medical assistant quickly readied a lancet and stuck Windora's finger, drawing a drop of blood to check her sugar on a hand-held meter.

"Doctor, it is 140," she said—that was high, not low. Megan had been right: Windora had been jolted by a massive stroke. One of the major blood vessels to her brain was blocked by a clot, and the flow of oxygen to the brain had slowed. The brain cannot tolerate being deprived of oxygen for very long, as the tissue supplied by the clotted artery begins to wither and liquefy, destroying brain cells. Windora's speech center was being strangled as we watched.

Clinical trials have demonstrated that stroke damage can be reversed by a rapid injection of powerful clot-busting drugs. If that does not work, doctors can enter the occluded blood vessel through a catheter and attempt to extract the clot. But every minute that passes lowers the chance of success. The clock was ticking. It was fortuitous that Windora had the stroke right in front of us, and our office building was connected to the hospital. The stroke team was standing by in the emergency room. As paramedics whisked Windora away, we had good reasons to hope.

In the emergency room a team of doctors, nurses, and technicians began the complicated ballet of procedures required to reverse a stroke. They raced through the stroke checklist with NASCAR precision. Windora's strength had been normal in the clinic minutes before, but now her right arm and leg flopped by her side, paralyzed. The stroke was progressing rapidly. The team sedated Windora and placed her on a ventilator. A brain scan confirmed the diagnosis. The physicians injected the clot-busting medication into an intravenous line in her

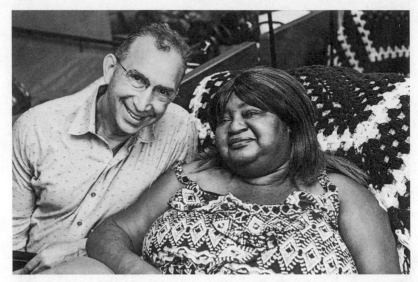

Windora and the author in 2016, after her stroke. Source: MHCooper Photography.

left forearm. For a moment, the room fell silent, other than the metronomic beeps of the heart monitor, as the team waited to see her response to the drug.

A few weeks before, the ever-cheerful Windora had been in the office talking with Megan about her illness, her hopes, and her fears. "The worst thing would be if I had a stroke where I still knew everything but could not speak," she had confided. Was this a premonition? Even in the best case, her worst fear seemed about to come true.

Only 30 percent of patients with a cerebral artery blockage respond to clot-busting medication. Those who do can experience miraculous recoveries. Windora was not one of them.

The stroke team members buzzed with energy as they activated Plan B: to suck the clot from the clogged vessel. This had been an experimental procedure until recently. Windora was wheeled to the nearby neurointerventional suite, which was laden with the latest technology. There the physician introduced a catheter into her groin, passed it up to the middle cerebral artery, and attempted to dislodge the clot. This got some of it out, and blood began to flow to the oxygen-deprived areas of Windora's brain. Windora's right leg began to move. Then her right arm moved—barely. A small success.

Eventually Windora would walk again, but the speech area of her brain was permanently damaged. She never spoke again—her worst fear. The last word she uttered had been my name.

Health Is a Human Right

Why did Windora Bradley get ill? Why do too many people like her die too soon in America? The answer is inequality caused by structural violence.

I became a primary care doctor to help people like Windora. I became an epidemiologist to understand and help change the social conditions that that deprive our communities and their residents of their vitality. Along the way, I began to see a side to America that is invisible to most middle-class and wealthy Americans—a side of America where the grind of racism and poverty steals years of life. I hope that this book will serve as a clarion call for fair-minded readers to join the fight against the structural forces that perpetuate inequality in America. It begins with the acknowledgment that health is a fundamental human right and not a commodity to be traded and sold in a marketplace. My own pursuit for health and social equity is inspired by a quote from Louis Pasteur engraved on a bronze plaque on a monument in a park across the street from County. It says, "One doesn't ask of one who suffers: What is your country and what is your religion? One merely says, you suffer, this is enough for me. You belong to me and I shall help you."[16]

STRUCTURAL VIOLENCE AND THE DEATH GAP

What we deal with in our work, quite apart from the extremes of geno-cide, is a variant of that: "Lives less worthy of life." When we say that the poor have a mortality rate that is multiple times the rate of the rich, when we say poor children die in our country and in the developing world at rates far higher than those of the better off, we are saying that we permit a condition which in effect says they are less worthy of life. We are sending this message because we let it happen, because we have social policies that almost assure that it will happen, and we let it happen stubbornly and continually.[1]

H. JACK GEIGER, MD

It might be difficult for some readers to conclude that structural vio-lence was a key causal factor in Windora Bradley's stroke. After all, Windora must bear responsibility for her self-care and health care out-comes, shouldn't she? But there are proximate causes and chronic—or structural—causes. Chronic diseases enact their toll over decades, obscuring deeper causes such as poverty, unemployment, and racism. Consequently, individual high-risk behaviors or biological consid-erations might confound the consideration of social and structural causes of death and dying. It is hard to tease out the social causes of illness from the individual drivers of illness and death when the time from disease onset to death is measured in decades, not days.

In addition, because doctors take care of patients who show symp-toms of individual diseases, it is hard to see patterns of illness and death unless they are analyzed in large numbers over time. It is only when you take a step back—add up disease and death numbers one by one, look at them by gender, income, race, and geography—do you realize that there are large gaps or inequalities in death rates. These gaps have been broadly called *health inequities*. When these gaps are the result of the health care system, they are called *health care inequities*. I prefer to use the term *death gaps* because it describes the actual outcomes of health inequity. People die prematurely because of inequity—that is, they experience higher death rates than would be expected in the absence of this inequity. A society where all people experienced the same mortality independent of race, gender, socioeconomic status, or geography would have no death gaps.

Why do these gaps or inequities in mortality exist? Doctors are trained to attribute disease to the poor habits, genetics, resistance, psychology, or poor physiology of their patients, because Western medicine focuses on the individual. Patients, too, attribute their diseases to their own failings. "I did not take care of myself," they say. "I did not eat right. I did not exercise. It runs in my family." Doctors and patients typically do not consider that the diseases they experience might be the embodiment of ills created by conditions imposed on the communities where the patients live.

We can see the difference more clearly in the case of a natural disaster like an earthquake, where social fault lines are exposed in seconds. In Haiti, a country whose people have long been victimized by structural violence, the aftermath of the 2010 earthquake was particularly deadly and brutal. I went to Haiti after that earthquake, and what I saw there helps provide insight on the impact of structural violence on chronic disease mortality in the United States.

Port-au-Prince Crumbles

On January 12, 2010, a 7.0 Richter-scale earthquake crumbled Port-au-Prince, Haiti, killing over 300,000 people. Most victims were trapped in the rubble, and many who were pulled from collapsed buildings died later from their injuries. In the course of the tectonic upheaval, 285,677 residences and 30,000 businesses were flattened, leaving more than a million people homeless in makeshift tent cities of sheets and cardboard that occupied every available square foot in the capital.[2] Yet a similar-scale earthquake in Oakland, California, in 1989 killed only 63 people and left 3,000 homeless.[3] Much of the difference in mortality between the two earthquakes was attributed to the more rigorous building codes in California, in addition to a well-developed emergency response infrastructure. Many of Haiti's buildings were constructed from concrete and cinderblock without earthquake precautions, leaving the populace at risk when the inevitable earthquake hit. Simply stated, Haiti was not prepared for a disaster of this scale.[4]

In ten seconds of similar earth-shattering devastation, one of the major differences between the United States and Haiti, the richest and the poorest countries in the Western Hemisphere, was exposed: place matters when it comes to life expectancy. There are death gaps between communities. When a natural disaster hits, the death gap is immediate, cataclysmic, and dramatic. Death comes swiftly and targets the poor and otherwise disadvantaged populations or neighborhoods in a graphic and heartbreaking manner.[5] If you happened to live in Port-au-Prince in 2010, you were much more likely to die from an earthquake than if you lived in Oakland in 1989. On a smaller scale, this truth also holds every day in rich and poor neighborhoods in cities like Chicago, Cleveland, Pittsburgh, and Philadelphia.

The high death rate in Port-au-Prince was caused by cumulative political, economic, cultural, and infrastructural failures. The structural failures, as well as the country's extreme poverty, were themselves caused by the complex and subordinate relationship Haiti has had with Western nations since earning its freedom in 1803, in the only successful slave rebellion in modern history.[6] The exploitation and impoverishment of Haiti in the two hundred years since its independence could not have occurred without the concentration of wealth at Haiti's expense in France, the United States, and other wealthy nations. One example is the $22 billion ransom demanded by France in 1825 as the price of Haitian freedom. This extortion was enforced by the international community at gunpoint as well as embargo, and even military occupation by the United States. Port-au-Prince became a city of extreme poverty and concentrated disadvantage, which in turn contributed, generations later, to the large death toll from the earthquake.

After the earthquake I joined a group of physicians and nurses in Haiti to provide medical relief. I was struck by the similarities between patients in Port-au-Prince and on the West Side of Chicago. Disease and death wear similar masks around the world. As doctors we are trained to meet an illness head-on, to wrestle with its physical, psychological, and social manifestations. Often our enemy is neither the disease nor the limits of our healing gifts but the structure of services and support in the community that keep treatment or palliation just beyond our reach. Rudolf Virchow described doctors as the "natural attorneys for the poor," because we are often placed in the role of personal advocates for our patients and their needs amid social, political, and economic structures that seem equally determined to deny them health.[7]

Dying of a Broken Heart

The error in blaming victims of structural violence for what happens to them is explicitly clear when we consider earthquake victims. No one can accuse earthquake victims of reaping the consequences of their own unhealthy behaviors.

Consider a patient I met two weeks after the earthquake hit. She survived the initial horror but now came to us with a related illness just as deadly as the quake itself. She was a bone-thin middle-aged woman who looked at least thirty years older than she was; the stresses of life in Haiti accelerate aging. Her face was deeply creased with wrinkles. Her brow and cheeks were covered with beads of sweat that gave her ebony skin an eggplant-purple sheen. Her sharp-edged face with bony cheekbones and chin could have been carved from a block of obsidian. She was half carried, half dragged, limp and listless to the hospital.

Our medical team was deployed to the Hospital of the State University of Haiti, or "the General," as it is known, Haiti's largest public hospital. Unfortunately, the hospital itself had suffered extensive damage during the quake. The nursing college had collapsed, trapping more than one hundred students and teachers inside. Many of the hospital

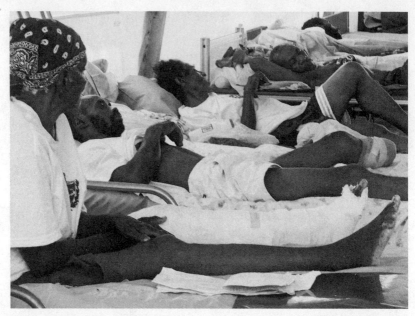

A tent hospital in Port-au-Prince, Haiti, after the 2010 earthquake. Source: author's personal collection.

buildings were uninhabitable, and the patients had been relocated into large tents donated by the international community. These tents were sixty feet long, open to the outside, and lined with row on row of cots filled with amputees, whose initial operations had been performed under grisly and unsanitary conditions. Now the stifling, humid air in the tents was pungent with a sickly sweet-and-sour aroma emanating from the infected stumps of these survivors, who languished while awaiting surgery. It looked more like a scene from a Civil War battleground than like one from a modern hospital.

They lugged the ill woman into a tent we had set up—an intensive care unit of sorts. She watched us with fear and distress as she gasped for air. Her neck veins were distended, and her ribs retracted as her body starved for oxygen. A nurse and I placed our arms underneath her and lifted her skeletal frame onto a cot, where she flopped like a rag doll, near collapse. She had been fine before the earthquake but in the aftermath had begun to get short of breath until each step left her exhausted. We examined her heart with an ultrasound and discovered that her heart muscle was floppy and pumped blood at a fraction of its normal capacity. She was not having a heart attack or suffering from hypertension. She seemed to have Takotsubo cardiomyopathy, a form of heart failure also known as "broken heart syndrome." The cause is unknown, but it has been associated with severe stress, such as the loss of a loved one or the emotional trauma associated with a natural disaster. Scientists believe that under sudden and extreme stress, the adrenal glands release a tsunami of adrenaline that overwhelms the nerve receptors and damages heart muscle in those who are susceptible. The heart muscle balloons into a flabby bag. As the heart loses its ability to pump, fluid backs up into the lungs, causing severe shortness of breath.[8]

We nursed this woman back to health, under the withering heat, with a combination of medications and oxygen. In a few days she was discharged, her "broken heart" now a bit improved. With lips pursed, she struggled to catch her breath while in one hand she clasped plastic bags filled with a rainbow of various medications—a one-month supply of American-made pills we had prescribed. With her free hand she clung to the bent neck of her grandson, who carried her piggyback from the hospital to the forlorn tent she now called home, among the city of tents in the middle of Port-au-Prince. My stomach sank as I saw her carted from the hospital grounds. Her brief stay in our makeshift overheated tent had likely been better than the conditions she'd experience in the tent city. It was hard to believe that her heart would survive there. Did she have clean water with which to take her medications? Would she survive the blistering heat? What would she do when her medications ran out? Most important, if she died, what would have been the true cause of her death? Heart failure or the strain caused by the earthquake, poverty, and unhealthy living conditions?

Death Certificates and Causes of Death

Cases of premature illness or death from post-earthquake Haiti seem remote from the disease and death experience in the United States. Yet the clinical conditions we treated in Port-au-Prince were similar to cases I have seen over the years in Chicago. But how do you make the leap from individual cases into a greater understanding of the death gaps across communities? It all starts with the death certificate.

For hundreds of years, modern societies have been recording deaths. In Europe and North America, death records were originally maintained by local churches. In 1639 the Massachusetts Bay Colony was the first American settlement to switch the responsibility for keeping these records from the churches to the courts.[9] By the late 1800s, European countries had begun to create central registries for recording deaths. The United States lagged behind until 1910, when its standardized death certificate was developed.[10]

It is the doctor's responsibility to record the chain of medical conditions leading to death, based on four categories. The first is the immediate cause of death: the precise disorder that directly preceded it. The second is intermediate causes: those conditions that created the immediate cause. The third is the underlying cause: the condition that set off the chain of events. Finally, the doctor is asked to list the patient's other ailments, even though they did not cause death. Eventually the certified cause of death becomes part of a long statistical trail, from the local physician to city and state health officials to the national death registry. It is then codified among the official vital statistics of the United States and other countries where the rates of death can be compared.

Over the years I have filled out hundreds of death certificates for my patients as my final act of caring. It was usually a poignant moment as I sat in the hospital admitting office with the name of the patient and the date and time of death already typed on the certificate by one of the clerks. Pen in hand, I took a moment to reflect on the life of my patient, the last time I saw him or her, what we talked about, family, quirks. Then I filled out the certificate and signed my name.

As simple as it sounds to document the cause of death, the chain of causation can be long, complicated, and incomplete. Sometimes the underlying or true cause of death is not apparent. If a smoker dies of lung cancer, the true cause might be cigarettes. But a doctor does not list cigarette smoking as a cause of death because smoking per se is not a disease. If my patient in Haiti with broken heart syndrome died, the cause of death on the death certificate would be heart failure. But what was the true underlying cause of death: the earthquake, poverty, or homelessness? The rules require the physician to list illnesses, not social conditions, as causes, even if poverty, racism, tobacco, pollution, and stress might be considered proximal causal conditions.

Inequality as a Cause of Death

I know that inequality is a cause of death, but not because I was taught about it in medical school or in residency training. You cannot find a chapter on inequality as a cause of death in any pathology textbook. And never once did I write "Inequity" as a cause of death on a death certificate. So if it is never recorded, how can we possibly measure or understand it?

There is a single measure of health that can be used to sum up health status and help us understand health inequality: life expectancy. Life expectancy is a number that takes into account every known cause of death in a population from infant mortality to deaths from epidemics like HIV and chronic diseases like heart disease. All rolled up into one number, life expectancy is a barometer of the health of a country or community. High life expectancy means better health status; low life expectancy means worse health status. Comparison of life expectancy rates between countries, counties, or communities allows us a peek at health inequality; since death rates from disease vary by location, so too does life expectancy. Just knowing that a death gap exists between two communities does not tell us *why* that gap exists, but it is a starting point to understand inequity in health and perhaps to begin to address it.

For example, life expectancy in Haiti in 2013 was 62.9 years. That was 186th worldwide—the lowest of any country in the Western Hemisphere. Life expectancy in the United States that year was 78.6 years, 51st in the world and the lowest among Western developed nations.[11] Therefore the death gap between Haiti and the US was 15.7 years (78.6 minus 62.9). In other words, Haitians—who do not have the same access to preventive measures, prenatal health care, societal safety measures, and health care—live on average almost sixteen years less than the average American. This overall death gap reflects specific gaps across a whole array of diseases and conditions, from infant mortality to deaths from cholera. This death gap cannot be attributed to biological or genetic differences between Haitians and Americans. Rather, it is the result of differences in political, economic, and social conditions and public health infrastructures.

In general, life expectancy in the world has risen over the past 150 years, with improved prevention and treatment of infectious diseases in the developing world and improved control of chronic diseases in the developed world.[12] We think of the United States as a very different society from Haiti, more developed, more sophisticated, more educated, with a better economy and health care system. Yet it would shock some people to know there are death gaps *between communities in the United States* that are greater than the one between Haiti and the United States.[13]

Life Expectancy Is a Priority

For over three decades, there has been increasing national recognition that death gaps between races and classes in the United States must be a public health priority. In 1990 the US Department of Health and Human Services created the "Healthy People 2000" campaign, with a goal to reduce health disparities by the year 2000. Subsequently, the "Healthy People 2010" goal was to eliminate health disparities by the year 2010.[14] Both campaigns have to be considered abject failures because while the income gaps, racial gaps, and geographic gaps in life expectancy have narrowed over time, they have not been eliminated. The gap between the US county with the highest life expectancy and the one with the lowest life expectancy is between thirty and thirty-five years, more than twice the gap between Haiti and the United States.[15] You can drive from Connecticut to rural Mississippi and watch three decades of life expectancy disappear. The gap in life expectancy in Chicago between the highest life-expectancy census tract and the lowest life-expectancy census tract is similar. Even as US life expectancy has marched steadily upward, those gains are largely benefiting those at the upper end of the income ladder. In fact, the death gaps between high socioeconomic groups and low socioeconomic groups have grown in the past three decades.[16]

Even more telling is the changing pattern of these regional, racial, and gender death gaps over time. In 1990 Drs. Colin McCord and Harold Freeman published a landmark paper in which they examined mortality rates by collecting causes of death from death certificates for residents of Central Harlem, a community that was 96 percent black and 41 percent below the poverty level. Their findings were startling. The age-adjusted mortality in Harlem was double that of the United States and 50 percent higher than that for all blacks in the United States. Most of the excess mortality occurred before the age of 65, and the causes included heart disease, cirrhosis, homicide, and cancer. They noted that the average black man in Harlem was less likely to reach the age of 65 than a man in Bangladesh.[17] Studies from Chicago, such as those done by Steven Whitman, also demonstrate increasing mortality gaps between black and white and between rich and poor residents between 1980 and 2010.[18]

Even worse, while racial mortality gaps were narrowing in some areas of the United States, they were increasing in Chicago and other urban areas. The authors of these studies called the prospects of achieving the Healthy People 2010 goals "bleak."[19] In fact, nationwide, racial gaps in deaths before the age of 65 increased from 1980 to 2000 after having decreased in the prior two decades.[20] The excess mortality is striking among black working-aged (16–64) residents of urban and rural high-poverty areas. Between 1980 and 2010 there was little decline in chronic disease mortality among these men and women in most areas, and in some instances there were increases. This suggests an entrenched burden of disease and unmet health care needs across many cities as well as rural areas.[21] While there have been some recent notable improvements in the overall life-expectancy gaps between whites and blacks, this is partly the result of growing mortality rates for whites—not the way we want to reduce disparity. But some of the improvement has been a result of some real progress for blacks (especially men), a result of decreasing cancer, homicide, and AIDS mortality between 1993 and 2013. Still, even with these improvements, there was a seven-year survival gap between white and black men in the United States as of 2013.[22]

Structural Violence and Premature Death

There is no deficit of startling statistics. One study found that a 16-year-old black boy on the South Side of Chicago had only a 50 percent chance of living to the age of 65.[23] The death rates were not much better for teens in Detroit or Harlem.

But they aren't just statistics, they're people. I give talks on health inequities every chance I get, hoping to get people as riled up as I am about this stain on American society. I found a photo of a young black man and pasted it into a PowerPoint slide. This kid is in all my talks. The unknown smooth-skinned teen smiles into the crowd as I ask, "Why does a black teen on the South Side of Chicago have only a 50 percent chance of living to 65? He's made it past the period of infant mortality and beyond childhood illnesses. So why are his odds no more than a flip of a coin?"

I have asked this question in many settings and to many audiences. A hand shoots up and the answer is always the same and always incorrect: "Violence," someone says.

Given the daily news reports of urban gunfights, it is not surprising that many people believe the major reason for the early death of urban working-age black men is homicide. While interpersonal violence contributes to the death gap in this age group, over half of the premature deaths in Chicago are from premature heart disease and cancer, diseases for which prevention, early detection, and treatment methods exist.

A 16-year-old black girl in the same neighborhood has only a somewhat better chance of living to 65 than the boy, while nationally more than 90 percent of 16-year-old girls will live to that age. And while urban poor white men and women in America have a greater chance of living to 65 than their poor black counterparts, they too experience death gaps relative to the overall white population, which has over an 80 percent chance of living to 65.[24] So yes, violence is the cause of death, but not interpersonal violence: this is structural violence.

Think about it another way. The average 50-year-old man in the same community as our 16-year-old will live eight years less than the average American white man. What are the implications of this? Families lose their older male role models in the prime of life, meaning that they often lose a source of wealth and perhaps wisdom. The unfairness is even greater than that. In such a community, large numbers of men and women, mostly poor, never reach the age to collect social security or Medicare, programs that they pay into during their working years. Those programs wind up funneling benefits upward, to the better-off people who survive to collect them—a perverted kind of welfare.

The deeper concern is how death gaps of such magnitude have settled into these communities. What is it about them that fosters ill health and premature mortality? Are the lifestyle choices of the residents of communities like Harlem responsible for the death gap between it and the Upper East Side? Have genetic and biological differences rendered the members of these urban communities more susceptible to disease? Or are these outcomes a result of structural violence: social, political, and economic arrangements, like racism and wealth inequality, that put individuals and populations in harm's way? And if so, what do we need to do to change them? If these political and economic arrangements are embedded in the organization of American society, *we can reverse them*.

There is an old tale about a country doctor. A man comes to his office with a broken leg. As the doctor repairs it he asks, "How did this happen?" The man replies, "I fell in a hole in the road." The next day, another man shows up at the doctor's office with a broken leg. Sure enough, as the doctor repairs the limb he discovers that this man had fallen into the same hole. The next day a third man comes to the office. He too has a broken leg; he had fallen into the hole as well. The next day the doctor grabs a shovel, leaves his office, and fills up the hole in the road.

This is the obligation of physicians. First we must treat our patients and relieve them of suffering and pain. But if we are to be the "natural attorneys" for our patients, we are also obligated to understand the true underlying causes of the death gaps that affect our communities. Only then can we begin to repair them.

3

LOCATION, LOCATION, LOCATION

Negro poverty is not white poverty. Many of its causes and many of its cures are the same. But there are differences—deep, corrosive, obstinate differences—radiating painful roots into the community, and into the family, and the nature of the individual. These differences are not racial differences. They are solely and simply the consequence of ancient brutality, past injustice and present prejudice.... For the Negro they are a constant reminder of oppression. For the white, they are a constant reminder of guilt.... Nor can these differences be understood as isolated infirmities. They are a seamless web. They cause each other. They result from each other. They reinforce each other.[1]

PRESIDENT LYNDON JOHNSON, 1965

"Location, location, location" are not only the three most important words in real estate; they are the three most important words in understanding health and wealth inequity in America. Location matters when it comes to health and longevity. To understand Windora Bradley's stroke or the Haitian woman's postearthquake heart disease in the context of structural violence, we first have to understand how low-life-expectancy neighborhoods have been formed and perpetuated in the United States in the last century, particularly in urban areas of the North and Midwest. Once we have established the importance of place in sickness, we will be able to explore how to build healthier communities.

This idea that neighborhood location matters when it comes to health and longevity is not new. In 1896 W. E. B. DuBois—the first black man to receive a PhD from Harvard, and a founder of the NAACP—studied the health conditions of the 40,000 blacks living in Philadelphia. He was one of the first social scientists to tie black-white health inequities not to biology but to the living conditions in various neighborhoods.[2] DuBois's study, the first of its kind, found that the economic and health status of the Philadelphia black community was rooted not in their heredity but in the environmental and social conditions imposed by the legacy of slavery and white supremacy. He wrote that because capitalism favored white workers over black workers, the economic life of the black community was continually destabilized. There were, he found, separate and unequal worlds of blacks and whites in economic and health terms. He concluded that the higher black death rates in 1896 Philadelphia were the result of living conditions, not race. DuBois's findings still hold true today.

The current racial makeup of many American cities and suburbs has its history in various influxes of blacks and Latinos, alongside the flight of whites from city centers.[3] Between 1910 and 1970 a "Great Migration" of six million blacks from fourteen southern states to northern, midwestern, and western cities changed the national character of the African American population from predominantly southern and rural to predominantly urban.[4] Prior to this migration only 7 percent of US blacks lived outside the South. By 1970 that had increased to 47 percent, with 80 percent of these migrants from the South living in urban areas.

In 1896 there were about 14,000 blacks living in Chicago. Migration expanded the population to 250,000 by 1930, but blacks were still only about 10 percent of Chicago's total population. From 1930 to 1960, the black population of Chicago quadrupled to almost one million, as more came in search of well-paying jobs.[5] Similar scenarios played out in New York, Philadelphia, Cleveland, Detroit, St. Louis, and other cities. Yet while the flow of southern blacks to northern and midwestern urban areas increased, neighborhood and housing options for these new migrants were limited to traditionally black areas within these cities. (In Chicago, for example, black immigrants were allowed to settle in only eleven of seventy-six community areas.) Restrictive covenants that prevented homeowners from selling property to members of certain racial, ethnic, and religious groups were legal in the United States until 1948.[6] Mob action, riots, and other forms of violent intimidation by angry whites also limited access to certain neighborhoods.

In the 1950s and 1960s, John McKnight was a community organizer with the Chicago Human Rights Commission and a leader in the era's fair-housing battles. Every summer night he traveled from neighborhood to neighborhood to observe and sometimes intervene in the race riots that inflamed Chicago during those years. "In any block where a black family moved in, there would be a big gathering of white people who would scream and yell in front of the house, throwing rocks and bricks through the windows," he recalls. "In some cases, they would light the wooden porches on fire. Night after night this would happen, to scare the blacks out. It was like a summer sport. The police stood at the end of the block doing nothing to intervene."[7]

Structural Violence in Mortgage Lending: "Redlining"

But it was not just incidents of racist urban violence that limited housing options for these migrants. Other forces of structural violence fueled neighborhood residential instability. Foremost were racist bank lending policies created and abetted by the US government and enforced by unscrupulous real estate agents, thugs, and the police. These lending policies had their roots in the Great Depression of the 1930s, when millions of mortgage holders defaulted and banks became wary of lending.

Homeowner lending by banks is an expression of trust, and if the lender does not trust the borrower, the property, or the neighborhood, it will not take the risk. In the United States, questions of lending trust have always been influenced by the borrower's race.[8] In 1933 Homer Hoyt, an economist at the University of Chicago, published a list of ten racial and ethnic groups, ranking them from positive to negative based on their perceived influence on property values. At the top of the list were Americans of English, Scottish, Irish, and Scandinavian heritage. At the bottom of the list, were Jews, Southern Italians, blacks, and Mexicans.[9]

Hoyt's racial rankings took on a new life when the federal government institutionalized "residential security maps" in 239 cities to classify the level of safety for real estate investments. Neighborhoods were assessed not only according to the age and condition of housing stock but also on the basis of their ethnicity, religion, economic status, and racial homogeneity.[10] These maps became guides for the private banking, real estate, and appraisal industries, carving out four types of neighborhoods. Predominantly white affluent suburbs on the outskirts of cities or other "desirable areas" were highlighted in green. Neighborhoods where blacks lived were outlined in cautionary red and considered the riskiest.[11]

McKnight uses the term *redlining* to denote the discriminatory lending practices of banks and the Federal Housing Authority (FHA) based on these maps. He tells how he discovered that the practice was widespread. "I remember going to the Federal Housing Authority in Indianapolis and asking the lead man there, 'Do you think there is redlining going on here?' The guy pulls down a wall map of Indianapolis and there was a big red line around all the black neighborhoods."[12]

If you wanted to purchase a home in a redlined neighborhood, the FHA would not guarantee the mortgage. In addition, FHA appraisal manuals were explicit in their promotion of residential segregation.[13] They instructed banks, which were typically white owned, to "prohibit the occupancy of properties except by the race for which they are intended."[14] The consequences of this racial profiling by banks, real estate agents, and the federal government were apparent in the results: between 1934 and 1962, $120 billion of federally guaranteed lending was devoted to creating mortgages for new housing, but less than 2 percent of it went to nonwhite families.[15]

Contract Selling, Blockbusting, and Panic Peddling

Denied access to FHA-guaranteed mortgages, blacks looking to buy homes could do so only by entering into private contracts with real estate speculators. These unscrupulous operators preyed on white homeowners' fears of real estate values plummeting due to the changing racial composition of their neighborhood. They would do things like hire black women to walk up and down the streets with baby strollers in white neighborhoods to give the impression that the neighborhood was changing. "It was an organized campaign of frightening people off," says McKnight. These "blockbusters," as they were called, bought houses on the cheap as they came up for sale, reselling them to African Americans at significantly higher prices. The terms of the contracts offered to blacks included maximum interest rates, all maintenance responsibilities, and the threat of eviction with total loss of investment for failure to pay at any time. Essentially, these contracts denied buyers many of the benefits traditionally associated with home ownership. Blockbusters waited for the buyer to miss a payment or some other pretext, repossessed the home, and started the process anew.[16]

Many families were evicted when they could not make the payments. Over time, this led to deterioration of the housing stock, paralyzed the housing market, lowered property values, and encouraged abandonment. Abandoned buildings were torched, often to collect insurance money, and empty lots proliferated, further destabilizing these neighborhoods.[17]

While the Fair Housing Act of 1968, the Home Mortgage Disclosure Act of 1975, and the Community Reinvestment Act of 1977 outlawed the worst of racially motivated lending practices, these laws are weak and have never effectively eliminated discrimination. Worse, by this time the neighborhoods had already undergone cataclysmic racial change driven largely by the white refusal to live alongside black people.

Between 1940 and 1980 thousands of urban neighborhoods across America flipped from all white to all black. However, out of 65,000 census tracts nationwide, only 10 transitioned from over 60 percent black to 60 percent white.[18] The rapid neighborhood turnover led one observer to quip that *integration* was no more than "a term to describe... the period of time that elapses between the appearance of the first Negro and the exit of the last white."[19] The end result was that rather than achieving any type of integration or stability, American urban neighborhoods became segregated and isolated.

I had a patient who purchased a house in North Lawndale as a middle-aged woman. In 2004 she was 104 years old, a four-foot-ten wisp of a woman with snow-white hair and a bright sparkle in her eyes. I made a house call to see her and her 98-year-old sister in their immaculate red brick bungalow, filled with the aromas of a half-century of home-cooked southern food.

"When we first moved in the neighbors were real nice," she recalled. In 1951 they had been the first black family in an all-white and Jewish neighborhood. But before long, "For Sale" signs were on every lawn, and soon her white neighbors fled.

"What were they running from?" I asked.

"Me, I guess!" she said with a grin, her eyes crinkling at the notion that her ninety-pound frame could sow that kind of fear.

But white flight was not just about simple prejudice. Racism is a powerful exploitative force. Speculators fueled white fears that the presence of black people would rob them of the wealth invested in their houses. The speculators in turn exploited the incoming black residents with usurious contracts and rents. It was often all about the money.

Neighborhood Disruption and Rapid Racial Turnover

A less appreciated factor in neighborhood segregation is the abandonment of urban centers by the nation's industrial and manufacturing giants. From 1950 to 1980, as the total black population in America's urban centers grew from 6.1 million to 15.3 million, industry fled to the suburbs along with white residents, leaving these newly segregated communities vulnerable to economic dislocation and joblessness.[20]

Between 1967 and 1987, manufacturing companies moved out of city centers, taking jobs and billions of dollars with them. Chicago lost 60 percent of its manufacturing jobs, or approximately 226,000. Detroit lost 51 percent, New York City 58 percent, and Philadelphia 64 percent.[21] As unemployment rates rose, the poor in these neighborhoods became poorer.[22] Between 1970 and 1980, two-thirds of the increase in the rate of extreme poverty was attributed to hypersegregated neighborhoods in New York, Chicago, Philadelphia, and Detroit.[23]

The flight of industry and the magnitude of job loss from North Lawndale during this period was mind-boggling. The community lost 69,000 jobs between 1968 and 1984. According to the *Chicago Reader*,

"By 1986, North Lawndale had 66,000 residents but only one bank and one supermarket. It also had 48 state lottery agents, 50 currency exchanges, and 99 liquor stores and bars."[24] That is, it didn't have jobs, but it did have a surfeit of exploitative businesses, further degrading the quality of life there. In 2016 there was still only one small supermarket in North Lawndale.

In addition to residential segregation and industrial abandonment, inner-city neighborhoods were isolated in three ways by the federal interstate highway system, which was first developed in the 1950s.[25] First, these highways provided avenues of flight for both white residents and industries. Second, construction of these highways was often designed to accelerate the demolition of "blighted" areas, which were often minority neighborhoods near city centers and white neighborhoods. Finally, local officials used some highways to create physical barriers between business districts, white residential neighborhoods, and nonwhite urban neighborhoods.[26] In Chicago, the Dan Ryan Expressway was built with federal highway dollars to link the southern suburbs with the commercial center.[27] Its eight lanes of macadam exacerbated the divide between burgeoning black Chicago to the east and white ethnic Chicago to the west.[28] Whether deliberately placed there or not, the expressway became a physical barrier that isolated black communities, accelerating their economic decline.

As these communities became ever more impoverished, as rates of health insurance decreased, and as doctors' offices and hospitals abandoned these neighborhoods, death gaps ensued. In Chicago, in the 1970s and 1980s fourteen neighborhood hospitals closed, many in redlined black neighborhoods.[29]

A Century of Hypersegrated Urban Neighborhoods

One immediate consequence of white flight was the creation of two kinds of American neighborhoods: those of concentrated poverty and disadvantage and those of concentrated wealth and advantage.[30] Neighborhoods of concentrated disadvantage are pockets of high poverty and high unemployment, and they are often racially segregated, with low life expectancy. Neighborhoods of concentrated advantage are low poverty and low unemployment, and while they too are often racially segregated, they have high life expectancy.[31] These neighborhoods did not develop in these ways by chance. Rather, they were direct consequences of discrimination, racist banking practices, and zoning regulations that kept blacks and low-income housing units out of these new suburbs. Whites disproportionately benefited from federal mortgage-guarantee programs. Developers encouraged them to buy houses in all-white suburbs. Low-interest guaranteed federal mortgages allowed them to accumulate wealth in these advantaged communities. A rising tide of wealth accumulation in the post–World War II years in the form of homeownership lifted the white middle class and all but bypassed black America.[32]

This is how structural violence works to benefit the lives of some at the expense of others. The neighborhood segregation and extreme poverty we see today are direct results of public and private policy decisions made decades before. There is no way to sugarcoat the conclusion. Neighborhoods of concentrated suffering, poverty, segregation, and low life expectancy developed across America because our political and economic power structures allowed wealth and well-being to be wrenched from them and given to others. These neighborhoods have persisted and even grown because policing, economic, trade, and taxation policies since the mid-1970s have been rigged to shift wealth to the advantaged few.

By 1990, 30 percent of blacks in the United States lived under conditions of intense segregation—neighborhoods that were over 90 percent black—with the rest inhabiting mostly black neighborhoods.[33] Routine social contact between races and classes became a rarity in such communities. Sociologist Douglas Massey has observed:

> Typical inhabitants of one of these ghettos are not only unlikely to come into contact with whites within the particular neighborhood where they live; even if they traveled to the adjacent neighborhood they would still be unlikely to see a white face and if they went to the next neighborhood beyond that, no whites would be there either.... Ironically, within a large, diverse, and highly mobile post-industrial society such as the United States, blacks living in the heart of the ghetto are among the most isolated people on earth.[34]

And this is true for better-off blacks as well. Even as the black middle class grew in the 1980s, its members relocated from high-crime black neighborhoods not to integrated middle-class neighborhoods but to more affluent segregated areas that were safer than their old neighborhoods, but not as safe as integrated neighborhoods.

We think about racial segregation as a phenomenon of black neighborhoods, when it is in fact an issue of white neighborhood organization. In parallel to black neighborhood segregation, almost 90 percent of suburban whites live in communities that are less than 1 percent black.[35] Many of these neighborhoods became segregated enclaves of concentrated advantage, unwilling to recognize that their advantages came at the expenses of others, to the detriment of the common good. In the twenty-first century Latino and Asian immigration has changed the nature of racial neighborhood makeup, as they move into traditionally white and mixed-race neighborhoods. Still, in 2010, 75 percent of whites in the United States still lived in all-white neighborhoods.[36]

Moreover, these inner-city neighborhoods remain the targets of unscrupulous operators, so their declines have not necessarily stopped, even today. In the first decade of the twenty-first century, the neighborhoods targeted by blockbusters in the 1950s were victimized again by unscrupulous subprime-mortgage lenders, who pushed fraudulent refinance and purchase loans on minority and low-income homeowners.[37] Urban areas largely in the Northeast and Midwest were hit hard (as were many areas across the United States), as these neighborhoods were already losing jobs and residents even when the national economy was strong. When the foreclosure crisis hit in 2007, the same neighborhoods were devastated once again.[38]

One might argue that neighborhood segregation in the post–civil rights era is a matter of personal choice and income inequality, but the facts suggest that racism is the driving force. Income inequality accounts for only 10 to 35 percent of segregation. In addition, only 17 percent of blacks say they prefer to live in black-only areas. And most whites say they would not live in black neighborhoods even if the percentage of blacks in the neighborhood was under twenty.[39] Racism created segregated neighborhoods, and racism maintains segregated neighborhoods of concentrated poverty.

Neighborhood Segregation's Many Gaps

The economic and health consequences of neighborhood segregation are enormous. Sociologists tracked the economic and health outcomes of a large cohort of black and white children raised after the civil rights movement. The black children had "substantially lower" incomes as adults than the white children—even when they were raised by parents with similar jobs and education levels. The key driver was the vastly different kinds of neighborhoods where the children grew up. The stark racial differences in neighborhoods have "been a primary mechanism for the reproduction of racial economic inequality in the post civil rights era."[40] The health outcomes of these groups are different as well, even after controlling for income and education.[41]

To appreciate the death gaps that this neighborhood dislocation and impoverishment caused, one need look no further than the South Side of Chicago. The University of Chicago, one of the best private universities in the country, sits in the Hyde Park neighborhood, a community that is flanked on the east by Lake Michigan and on the west by Washington Park, a masterpiece of landscape architecture with grassy meadows, oak trees, bike paths, and playing fields. The tree-lined streets of Hyde Park are alive with a diverse group of professors, students, and professionals. Hyde Park is also home to some of the best health care in the United States, courtesy of the University of Chicago Hospital, a top academic medical center whose steel-and-glass tower peers over Washington Park. Hyde Park is a neighborhood of concentrated advantage. Hyde Park is also a racially integrated community, one of the few such neighborhoods in the region. The life expectancy in Hyde Park in 2010 was 83 years, in the top quartile of Chicago community areas.[42]

Just west of Washington Park is a neighborhood of the same name. Cross that half-mile stretch of manicured green space and you might think you'd crossed from the Earth to the Moon. Squat, run-down buildings hug the drab treeless streets. Many storefronts are covered with steel gates or boarded up. Bedraggled men loiter on the corner of Garfield Boulevard and Michigan Avenue—not the gleaming, high-rise-lined Magnificent Mile of North Michigan Avenue, but its dreary four-lane South Side stepchild, dotted with check-cashing businesses and empty lots. The population of Washington Park is almost 100 percent African American and uniformly low income. Washington Park is a neighborhood of concentrated disadvantage. In 2010 the average life expectancy of a Washington Park resident was 69 years, placing it in the lowest quartile of Chicago communities and on par with Harlem in 1979–81.[43] The only hospital in Washington Park is Provident Hospital of Cook County, once the city's sole black-owned private hospital; in more recent years it has become a diminished outpost of the region's public hospital system, plagued by funding shortages and limited services.[44]

If Hyde Park were a country, it would be ranked second in the world with regard to life expectancy, equivalent to Spain. Washington Park, on the other hand, would be ranked 141st, tied with Iraq.[45] Spain is 2,600 miles away from Iraq. Yet Hyde Park is cheek by jowl with Washington Park, separated by a small patch of green. You can walk the half-mile from Hyde Park to Washington Park and watch fourteen years of life evaporate.

These neighborhood death gaps are not just a Chicago phenomenon. Across the United States there are graphic geographic gaps in survival between neighborhoods that sit nearly side by side. In 2003 in Cleveland, life expectancy in the suburban neighborhood of Lyndenhurst was 88, while eight miles closer to downtown, in the neighborhood of Hough, life expectancy was 64 years—a twenty-four-year plummet. In New Orleans, life expectancy hovers at 80 years in the wealthy neighborhood of Navarre but drops to 55 years in the French Quarter, three and a half miles away.[46]

Dead, White, and Blue

And the death gap is not just a problem for urban blacks, though they bear the worst brunt of it. In the United States there are eight distinct subgroups that vary greatly in life expectancy based on geography and race, ethnicity, and poverty.[47] At the top, with the highest life expectancies, are Asian Americans and northern white Americans, followed by white Middle America. At the bottom of the ladder are Appalachian

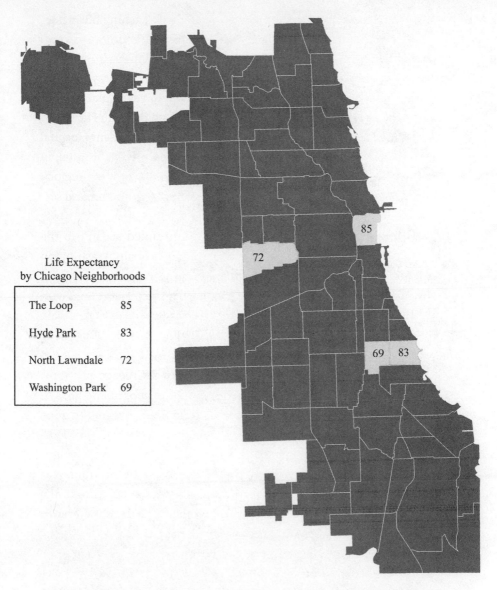

Life Expectancy
by Chicago Neighborhoods

The Loop	85
Hyde Park	83
North Lawndale	72
Washington Park	69

In Chicago, life expectancy can vary greatly depending on the neighborhood of residence. An affluent downtown neighborhood, the Loop, has median incomes of over $80,000 and the highest life expectancy in Chicago at 85 years old. Just five miles from the Loop, North Lawndale residents, 91 percent of whom are African American, have a median income of less than $25,000 and one of the lowest life expectancies at 72 years. In racially diverse Hyde Park, life expectancy is 14 years longer than in Washington Park to the west, where residents are almost entirely African American. Source: *New York Times*, 2015.

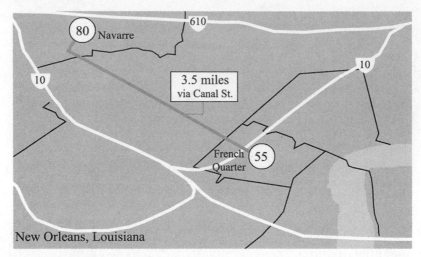

New Orleans, Louisiana

Across the United States, there are geographic gaps in life expectancy among neighborhoods that are in proximity to each other. In New Orleans, in a 3.5-mile drive from Navarre to the French Quarter, life expectancy drops 25 years. Source: Democracy Collaborative 2015 and Robert Wood Johnson Foundation.

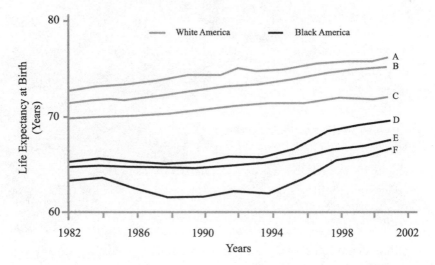

This graph shows the variance in life expectancy taking into account different combinations of socioeconomic, racial, and geographic variables. The six regional groupings are (A) white Americans in central-western United States, (B) whites in Middle America, (C) whites in Appalachia, (D) black Americans in suburban and metropolitan areas, (E) blacks in the rural South, and (F) blacks in the inner city. Source: "Eight Americas: Investigating Mortality Disparities across Races, Countries, and Race—Counties in the United States," *PLOS Medicine*, 2006.

whites, Native Americans, non-inner-city black Americans, rural black Americans, and, at the bottom, black Americans who live in distressed inner-city neighborhoods.[48] Clearly, premature mortality affects African Americans greatly, but they are not the only victims. The living and health conditions of Native Americans on reservations in the West leave them with reduced life spans as well.[49] The average male life expectancy on the Pine Ridge Reservation in South Dakota was reported to be 48 years, among the lowest in the Western Hemisphere.[50]

There are clusters of whites in the United States with high premature-mortality rates. And those rates are on the rise. Since 1999, low-income poorly educated whites from ages 25–34 and 45–54 have been dying at unprecedented rates, largely from suicide, alcoholic liver disease, and drug overdose. These rates have largely reversed life-expectancy gains resulting from improved treatment of chronic diseases in these groups.[51] They live in towns and cities where factories and mines have been shuttered by multinational corporations. Well-paying jobs have evaporated here just as they did in inner-city Chicago.

"There are large numbers of people who never get established in the economy, who live outside family relationships and are on the edge of poverty," sociologist Mark Hayward told the *New York Times*.[52] "Poverty and stress are risk factors for misuse of prescription narcotics," he said. And that drug use leads to premature death.

Had the death rates in these groups of whites continued to drop as they had in the twenty years prior to 1999, 500,000 fewer lives would have been lost between 1999 and 2013, equal to the number of deaths caused by the AIDS epidemic through 2015. The causes of death and concurrent plummeting rates of self-reported "well-being" suggest that this population group is experiencing unprecedented midlife stress.

The rocketing death rate among young white adults and steadily falling death rates among young black adults overall have shrunk the death gap between these groups by two-thirds. But this reduction is largely driven by rising white deaths.[53]

As one example, consider the living conditions in McDowell County, West Virginia, where the life expectancy of the white population is similar to that of people in Iraq. McDowell County was once home to thriving coal-mining operations. But as the demand for mineworkers dropped, the living conditions and the life expectancies in McDowell County began deteriorate. Now, the living conditions and disease burdens in McDowell County are like those seen in Windora Bradley's neighborhood of Chicago, with excessive rates of obesity, smoking, heart disease, and diabetes.

There is another twist to this story. For the wealthy, location has no impact on longevity. But for the poor, like Windora, geography is destiny. Where the poor call home can be a matter of life and death. This is true in neighborhoods across the country. It has long been known that individuals with higher incomes can expect to live up to fifteen years longer than those at the bottom and that the relationship is not simply between rich and poor but operates along an income gradient. The top 1 percent are not only richer—they are healthier.[54] But for the poor, geography also has a legacy impact on longevity. Poor residents of certain cities live up to five years longer than the poor in others. The specific reasons why some of the poor live longer are unclear but likely have to do with the structures that govern day-to-day life such as public health policies that influence health habits and the strength of the health-care safety net.[55] This fact gives great hope that these seemingly intractable life-expectancy gaps can be reduced.

Third World Conditions within a Superpower

It's critical to note, however, that white poverty is not concentrated like black poverty, because whites have so many more options for residential mobility than blacks do. Not surprisingly, cities like Chicago, New Orleans, and Cleveland, whose residents experience large death gaps, also rank high on a dissimilarity index: a measure of racial segregation that represents the percentage of a racial group that would have to move out of a neighborhood for the group to be perfectly integrated in a city or metropolitan area. The higher the number (between 0 and 1), the greater the level of racial segregation. Chicago ranks as the fifth-most-segregated city in America out of 318, with a dissimilarity index of 0.84, meaning that 84 percent of Chicago's black population would need to move from their neighborhoods into white neighborhoods in order for full racial integration to be achieved.[56]

Take a step back and add up all the statistics about black America, and the death gaps begin to make sense. Aggregate all the data and there is just one inescapable conclusion. Black America is a very oppressed and fragile state embedded within a white superpower. The black unemployment rate would rank Black America among the worst thirty countries in the world for employment. The poverty level in Black America is higher than that in Iraq. The median black income is a tad above that of the average Palestinian.

Black America lags thirty places behind the United States as a whole on the Human Development Index, which measures things like health, life expectancy, education, and income. The imprisonment rate of black Americans is the highest in the world, and the homicide rate resembles that of Haiti. On the Fund for Peace's Fragile State Index, Black America would be on the "High Alert" list.[57] If Black America were a country, we would have to send in foreign aid. This disastrous scenario could not exist if structural violence did not sustain it.

In his 1963 "I Have a Dream" speech, Martin Luther King Jr. said, "We cannot be satisfied as long as the Negro's basic mobility is from a smaller ghetto to a larger one."[58] But in Chicago and around the United States, that's exactly what happened, with dire consequences for health.

4

PERCEPTION IS REALITY

This is our basic conclusion. Our nation is moving towards two societies, one black and one white—separate and unequal. Segregation and poverty have created.... a destructive environment totally unknown to most white Americans. What white Americans have never fully understood— but what the Negro can never forget—is that white society is deeply implicated in the ghetto. White institutions created it, white institutions maintain it, and white society condones it.[1]

KERNER COMMISSION REPORT, 1967

While it's clear that historically structural violence fueled the creation of highly segregated, high-poverty black and Latino communities across the United States, present-day racial and ethnic bias also perpetuates poverty and ill health in these neighborhoods.[2] This form of structural violence fuels continued racial and economic segregation in America. The conditions in high-mortality neighborhoods of concentrated poverty are remediable and reversible, but only if we are able to cultivate greater empathy than what we tend to see in American society today. Because only when we stand in pragmatic solidarity with the people suffering from poverty, illness, and early death can we begin to reverse the conditions of misery in which they live. This begins with empathy and compassion.

The Empathy and Wealth Gap

There is an empathy gap in America. Members of communities of concentrated affluence have lost their sense of community responsibility for those living in concentrated poverty. An unparalleled proportion of the national income now goes to the top 20 percent of Americans. They have accumulated wealth at the expense of the poor and have dissociated themselves from responsibility for their well-being. These people have little need of national health insurance, income support programs, public education, and public health programs. They also have little use for public policies (including taxes) that limit the inheritance of deprivation from parents to children. Their wealth and political power give them unprecedented ability to shape public policies that favor the rich at the expense of the poor.

Tax laws that favor the wealthy over the poor and middle class, for example, redistributed billions of dollars of American wealth into the pockets of the rich. In 1955 the 400 richest Americans paid over 51 percent of their income in federal taxes. In 2007 that rate was a little under 17% percent.[3] Tax cuts for the wealthy and corporations cost the US Treasury $700 billion between 2001 and 2008. Meanwhile, safety-net programs were slashed to accommodate these tax cuts. In addition, trade policies exported millions of well-paying American jobs overseas. As a result of these policies, two-thirds of the gains in income in the United States between 2002 and 2007 flowed to the top 1 percent of households.[4] The Great Recession of 2008 only widened the chasms between the rich and others. By 2007, federal tax policy allowed the top 1 percent to gain a larger share of income than at any time since 1928.[5] The rise in income of the top 20 percent of earners now far outstrips that of the lowest 20 percent, who have experienced almost no real income growth since 1975.[6] Recently the Federal Reserve Bank surveyed Americans about their economic health. When asked how they would pay for a $400 emergency, a full 47 percent said they would have to borrow the money or sell something to raise it.[7]

One might be led to believe that higher taxes in the mid-twentieth century were a damper on economic growth. But the post–World War II economic boom was marked by high income taxes and a strong social infrastructure. These taxes were reinvested into the American people. Veterans went to college for free. College tuitions at public institutions were affordable. The interstate highway system enhanced commerce. Families could buy homes with government support. The Medicare and Medicaid programs provided health care for the elderly and poor, respectively. Incomes grew at about the same rate for the rich and everyone else during this period.[8]

If we are serious about transforming high-mortality neighborhoods like Windora's into healthier places, it will require large investments and wealth redistribution back into these communities. This will require the top 20 percent of Americans to use their disproportional political power to relinquish some of their wealth through taxation. This requires understanding that the inequality in wealth accumulation has occurred to the detriment of others.

The experience of personal suffering is not easily reduced to a graph or a statistic. It is real people who are ill and dying because of inequality. My work as a doctor requires me to witness travails and tribulations that people like Windora and her family have endured. But the lives of the poor rarely intrude into the consciousness of the affluent, even when the distribution of wealth to the wealthy is partly responsible for the suffering. Just as place matters when it comes to illness and premature death, community matters when it comes to improving health. Any community solution to illness caused by poverty or racism requires members of communities of concentrated affluence to witness the suffering of their fellow citizens in neighborhoods of concentrated poverty. And to support policies that might mitigate suffering even if it comes at their personal expense.

The Perception Gap and the Empathy Gap

Niraj is a Houston-based physician I met at a conference where I spoke about health care inequity. He told me that his comfortable, well-off friends and neighbors were both derisive of and dismissive toward the plight of the poor, disadvantaged, and mostly black residents of inner-city neighborhoods of Houston.

"They have no empathy for the poor," Niraj confided. "They blame them for their misfortune." He continued: "You know, 30 percent of the Houston population is uninsured." Moreover, he said, "those who *are* insured and working as plumbers or policemen are just one illness away from medical bankruptcy. When I tell my friends, they scoff. They say things like 'Well, they should have thought about this when they became a plumber instead of a doctor or a lawyer.'"

Communities like Niraj's have become gated enclaves of economic privilege. Such privilege stems from growing income inequality. Increasingly, researchers believe that growing income gaps have contributed to the widening of the American death gaps.[9] But there is another gap that contributes to the death gap—something I call the "perception gap." Residents of better-off communities have abandoned communities of concentrated disadvantage, first, by the act of fleeing the neighborhoods; second, by withdrawal of political support for policies that might lift these neighborhoods from poverty; and third, by endorsing negative perceptions that blame rather than empathize with the residents of these neighborhoods. Such perceptions contribute to the persistence of poverty, and thus to the death gap in America's downtrodden neighborhoods.[10]

Many privileged US communities are in suburbs or exurbs of major metropolitan areas; a half-hour drive can reveal income and death gaps as extreme as any in the world. Like Niraj's neighbors, some residents of these communities express indifference to or outright antagonism for the plight of the poor. They believe the choices that poor people make mire them in poverty and despair. While there are many white disadvantaged neighborhoods across the United States, the most disadvantaged communities in major metropolitan areas tend to comprise African Americans, Latinos, and Asians, adding a racist dimension to the critiques. Part of the perception gap arises from the fact that decades of economic and racial segregation have eliminated opportunities for routine interactions that could humanize relationships between members of disparate racial and economic communities. Racism fueled segregation, which fuels perception and empathy gaps in a vicious cycle.

But where do these negative perceptions come from, and how do they maintain their surface validity?

The American Millstone

In 1986 the *Chicago Tribune* ran a series of articles titled "The American Millstone."[11] They described the downward spiral of North Lawndale and the rise of a "permanent underclass," a migrant minority that had carved out a place for itself in the basement of the American dream. They portrayed a group of black people who had become hopelessly trapped, unable to break the chain of poverty and despair.

I spent a decade at Mount Sinai Hospital in North Lawndale and immersed myself in providing medical care to the members of that community. While I knew the history of the community—its Eastern European and Jewish roots, the black migration, the redlining, the blockbusting, the white flight, the flight of industry, the devolution of the neighborhood—I was not aware that the conditions were as dire as the *Tribune* reported. I knew Lawndale had a network of churches, community health centers, some excellent schools, and, of course, Mount Sinai Hospital, the largest employer in the community.

Yet it was difficult to quarrel with the gist of the *Tribune*'s critique. Lawndale was a neighborhood with high poverty, high unemployment, high crime, and high mortality.[12] That is as true, or even more so, today. If you drive through Lawndale, the disorder is apparent, much like what I described in Washington Park. Plastic bags, tossed by the famous Chicago winds, tumble ghostlike across broken cement. Graffiti is spray-painted on boarded-up storefronts and announces the buildings' abandoned status as well as the street gang that works the block. Of the buildings that remain inhabited, some of the windows are barred, others are broken. What few businesses there are tend to be fish joints, car-repair shops, beauty shops, and storefront churches. Rubble-filled empty lots stipple the streetscape, interspersed with brick and stone two- or three-flat homes. People, mostly African American men, gather on street corners and empty lots to kibitz. North Lawndale seems on first glance to be a "bad" neighborhood, riddled with crime, disinvestment, and ill health.[13]

But is everything as it seems?

Broken Windows Theory and Racial Bias

Debates about the meaning of urban disorder and good and bad neighborhoods have raged since the early publications of the Chicago School of urban sociology in the 1920s and 1930s.[14] Sociologists noted the "incivilities" and high crime rates associated with disordered neighborhoods and classified neighborhoods as "good" or "bad" based on the presence of disorder.[15] As increasing numbers of minorities and immigrants spilled into urban neighborhoods, observers began to conflate diversity and disorder, so that neighborhoods that were home to large numbers of minorities were considered "bad" by association.[16]

Those debates about disorder and crime were antecedents for a popular contemporary theory about community disorder and "bad" neighborhoods: the broken windows theory.[17] The link between broken windows and crime seems at first glance direct and logical. A lot is abandoned. Weeds grow in the front lawn. A window is shattered. A porch needs repair. Elders neglect to reprimand unruly children. Middle-class families begin to move out, leaving behind individuals who either cannot escape or do not want to leave. There are public acts of disrespect, drinking in public, loud music playing, and fights. These small acts of "incivility" accumulate. Petty criminals interpret these signs of community apathy as encouragement, since they believe the chance of getting nabbed for criminal behavior is low. Crime grows in the neighborhood. First it is minor crime. A bicycle or purse is snatched. Major crimes follow. The neighborhood is shattered by assault and arson, mayhem and murder. Residents steer clear of the streets. When they must go outside, they do so in stealth, heads down, hands in pockets. Windows are barred. Mothers shoo their children home after school. Children become indoor captives. Television is the substitute for outdoor play. The conventional neighborhood no longer exists. What is left is a geographic desert of disorder susceptible to criminal deterioration. A disordered neighborhood becomes a "bad" neighborhood. And often, a bad neighborhood is a neighborhood with poor health outcomes and low life expectancies.[18]

Does the broken windows theory help explain the sixty years of

deterioration in North Lawndale? The surface plausibility is very at-
tractive. It seems to explain neighborhood decline, and it prescribes
a "law and order" approach to rectify it. Beginning in the late 1980s
but especially through the 1990s, the theory was widely adopted, in-
stigating changes in policing and fueling the draconian War on Drugs.
These theories drove policing policies well into the twenty-first century.
As an example, in 2006 Mayor Thomas M. Menino ordered Boston
police to "crack down" on petty crime. Policeman broke up loud par-
ties and public drinking, and became tough on littering. At a press
conference, the mayor announced, "Today we are addressing what may
sometimes appear to be smaller issues... but we know that these kinds
of community disorder issues are the precursors to the violent crimes
that may follow."[19] The New York Police Department relied heavily on
an offshoot of the broken windows theory, called "Stop and Frisk,"
a policing policy that in 2011 precipitated almost 700,000 incidents
involving New Yorkers, 91 percent of whom were racial minorities. Due
to public and court pressure, "Stop and Frisk" incidents were reduced
to 50,000 by 2013. The New York City crime rate did not increase.[20]

Implicit Bias and Neighborhood Decline

Not everyone believes in the broken windows theory, and its logic has
not always been borne out.[21] Harvard sociologist Robert Sampson is a
broken windows skeptic. He asked: what if it is not disorder itself but
the *perception* of disorder that tarnishes a neighborhood's reputation?[22]
Walk down the south side of the Seine in Paris, and long stretches of the
embankments are decorated with vast expanses of multicolored graffiti.
However, against this background, couples stroll hand in hand in the
twilight hours along the river. Why is this graffiti perceived as "color-
ful" or "edgy" while graffiti in North Lawndale or inner-city Houston
evokes crime, fear, and urban decline? What makes one neighborhood
feel "bad" and another "good"? Could it be that "disorder" is contextu-
ally shaped by social conditions?[23]

Mounting evidence suggests that human cognition relies in part on
brain processes that operate quickly and create snap judgments that
when tested against evidence might not hold. The basic machinery for

snap judgments was present in the brains of our distant ancestors, and the same structures are still found in our brains today.[24] These cognitive processes operate below that part of the brain that weighs data and evidence before acting—deliberate "cold" reasoning. Social psychology literature has shown that cultural and racial stereotypes, called "implicit bias," operate on this level and persist even in the absence of personal racist animus.[25] For example, studies confirm that young North American children, both black and white, on average assign more negative adjectives to drawings of black faces and more positive adjectives to drawings of white faces.[26] Consider also the experiment in which subjects were told to shoot armed men and not unarmed men. Subjects, black or white, were more likely to make the correct decision to shoot an armed man if he was black rather than white.[27]

When my mother-in-law was helping my wife and me select our first home in Oak Park, Illinois, a mixed-race suburb just west of Chicago, she saw a black man walking down the street. "I would never live in a neighborhood with blacks," she advised.

Just the visual cue of a black man on a stroll down a tree-lined suburban cul-de-sac was enough to change her impression of our house from a good buy to perhaps an undesirable risk. Could unconscious, collective, and implicit bias be driving our perceptions of which neighborhoods are "good" and "bad"? Are these same biased perceptions motivating Niraj's suburban neighbors?

Perceptions, Not Reality

Robert Sampson studied neighborhood perceptions in his Project on Human Development in Chicago Neighborhoods (PHDCN). The PHDCN began as a criminology study and soon morphed into an interdisciplinary sociological, epidemiological, demographic, and geographical project involving cohort studies, community surveys, and street observations, among other undertakings. One aspect of it was designed in part to test the validity of the broken windows theory and to understand the links between the physical and social structures of neighborhoods and other characteristics such as juvenile delinquency, crime, and health.[28] Studies in the PHDCN included interviews with residents, panels with community leaders, and a longitudinal cohort study of more than 6,000 children. Researchers also mounted cameras on SUVs to record neighborhood activity, graffiti, and broken glass across 22,000 streets in 350 neighborhoods. They then rated the neighborhoods on the degree of disorder from these findings. Through the examination of juvenile delinquency, adult crime, teenage sexuality, substance abuse, homicide and mental health, Sampson was able to link evidence from neighborhood environments in Chicago to their effects on individuals within these communities, including health.[29]

Sampson discovered that actual signs of physical and social disorder in a neighborhood were much less influential in shaping people's perceptions of disorder than the racial, ethnic, and class composition of that neighborhood. Residents perceived more disorder in predominantly black than in predominantly white neighborhoods, even when the observable evidence was identical. Neighborhood residents of all races perceived more disorder in mostly black and poor neighborhoods than in equivalently disordered white neighborhoods. When whites, blacks, and Latinos lived in the same neighborhood and were exposed to the same conditions, whites were likely to perceive greater disorder than blacks and Latinos did.[30]

Contrary to the broken windows theory, real disorder did not predict neighborhood decline. However, race- and poverty-conditioned perceptions of disorder in a neighborhood were powerful and durable predictors of future neighborhood decline. When such racial perceptions are widely shared across social networks, they become "sticky"— that is, they become even more predictive of a neighborhood's downward dive, especially if it is nonwhite. If it is widely perceived that a neighborhood is bad, it will become bad.

Research shows that Americans hold steadfast beliefs that connect blacks, Latinos, and immigrant groups to crime, violence, and disorder.[31] Each time a community gets more African American residents and white residents migrate, it leads to further stigmatization, crime, and civic withdrawal, further deepening poverty and hypersegregation.[32] As Sampson concludes, "Race is a mode of perceptual categorization people use to navigate themselves through a murky, uncertain world."[33] Because race is such a significant factor in decisions about where to live, where to shop, and where to send children to school, communities of color become permanently marked—and trapped in poverty—for the "crime" of being black or brown.[34] Neighborhoods that adjoin stigmatized poor black communities are more likely to get stereotyped, stigmatized, and racially segregated themselves, leading to blocks upon blocks of "locked-in" hypersegregation and poverty. The same is not as true of white neighborhoods where poverty is more interspersed and diluted.[35]

The United States is filled with these poverty traps. Given the country's urbanization, its stark juxtaposition of advantaged and disadvantaged communities across urban landscapes, and its historic legacy of discrimination in housing and education, it is no surprise that some of the most stigmatized and high-mortality poor neighborhoods are inner-city and African American.[36] These areas are defined by, and victims of, a combination of structural racism and geography: placeism.

Yet these neighborhoods are not static. People move in and out of them all the time. Sometimes this can lead to mixing, if not by race then at least by class, at least briefly. This can have a positive effect on a community. Poor people in neighborhoods that include more affluent individuals are less likely to drop out of school and score better on some health measures than poor people who are surrounded by poverty—probably because the neighborhood affluence raises the ability of all its members to succeed.[37] Think about the life of a poor child who is raised in an affluent suburb. Her school choices are different. She might receive more attention in the classroom. She may have more exposure to healthy foods and exercise options. Perhaps through day-to-day contact with classmates and friends she has more exposures to the breadth of possibilities that life offers. But too often in America, children born into poverty live among other poor children and families.

Stuck in Place

True upward mobility is a myth in US society, especially for black people. Eighty percent of blacks and 70 percent of whites living in high-poverty neighborhoods stay stuck in those neighborhoods for generations. But whites overall are three times more likely than blacks or Latinos to move from a high-poverty area to a low-poverty neighborhood, while blacks are four times more likely than whites to experience downward mobility into worse neighborhoods.[38]

The fact is neighborhoods choose people, based on their circumstances; people do not choose neighborhoods, and this has negative consequences for health and welfare. When populations are geographically, socially, and economically isolated, regardless of race and ethnicity, they have higher disease and mortality rates.

Windora Bradley's Neighborhood

Windora Bradley had no degree in sociology. She was not a doctor. But the year before her stroke robbed her of her voice, we discussed her neighborhood and its impact on health. She had come in to see me for a checkup. I saw by the red spider-web of blood vessels that crisscrossed the whites of her eyes and the crow's feet of wrinkles surrounding them that she was worn out. Windora always had a positive spin on her travails, but not today. Today she was fretting.

"I was up all night in the Northwestern Emergency, with Darrell. His sugar was 800 and they gave him fluid until it came down to the 400s."

I knew that Windora's parents and one sister were dead from diabetes, and she had it as well. Now Darrell, her partner for almost two decades, had it. Blood sugars as high as Darrell's were deadly—a medical emergency.

"He don't have no insurance, and he needs a primary care doctor. He did not want to go to the doctor because he was afraid and he did not have money to pay," she said, frowning. Creases of worry appeared around her lips, and her shoulders slumped. Many times she had rationed her own medications because even with insurance her copayments for them were sometimes too much for her to manage on her small school-system pension (which substitutes for social security rather than supplementing it). This rationing made the medications less effective.

She talked about her neighborhood, one of Chicago's hot spots for crime and high mortality. "We all live together on my street. My neighbor is Mexican. There are Puerto Ricans across the street, and above them a black family. We all stick together. They used not to have any grocery stores, only little corner stores—I call them candy stores. They weren't nothing. And they only sold starchy junk foods and candy, no fruit or vegetables. So when the children were hungry we fed them sugars and starches. We knew it was not good for them, but we did not have any other choices." She recalled how she and her neighbors had petitioned the alderman to bring a real grocery store into the neighborhood a few years prior. "Now we can get vegetables and fruit," she said, "but most of the time we do not have the money to buy it." She shrugged.

Her sister and brother-in-law lived in a suburban neighborhood where they could walk safely. She contrasted this to her own neighborhood. "I don't let any of the grandchildren go outside or even sit on the front porch. It's not safe."

She knew this from painful experience. One Easter, Windora's eight-year-old granddaughter was playing in the alley down the street from the house. Two teenage gang members ran by, guns blazing. Windora's granddaughter was caught in the crossfire and collapsed in a pool of blood on the pavement, the screams of her playmates ricocheting off the brick walls as the color drained from her face. She was dead within minutes. After the murder, Windora limited outside activity. Everyone was ordered to stay inside, even Darrell. The cycle of inactivity, obesity, poor food choices, and stress created the perfect environment for diabetes to strike once again, this time at Darrell. Windora chuckled and shook her head,

"Darrell don't believe that. Darrell says he caught diabetes from me!"

Empathy and Death Gaps

How can we have anything but empathy for Windora and her family? It is not her fault that her neighborhood is unsafe. It is a cruel irony that even as structural violence in neighborhoods like Windora's creates poor health outcomes in their residents, too many people—like Niraj's gated-community neighbors—blame those residents themselves for the higher death rates that are killing them. This lack of empathy itself

kills in three ways. First, as Robert Sampson's experiments demonstrate, negative perceptions of poor neighborhoods perpetuate poverty,
accelerate neighborhood decline, and thus increase death rates there.[39]
Second, because the wealthy have more access to the political process
than the poor, they are more likely to influence policies that support
their interests at the expense of policies that might raise the lowest
levels of American society out of poverty. And third, when a subset
of influential Americans withdraws from investment in the common
good, their perception becomes a self-fulfilling prophecy, passed on
from generation to generation. The lack of social interactions among
members of different economic and ethnic communities exacerbates
the perpetuation of negative stereotypes.

If we hope to close poverty and death gaps, we need to apply the
knowledge and financial success strategies of affluent communities in
poor (mostly black and brown) neighborhoods. This will require compassion and empathy. But compassion and empathy are not enough.
There need to be structural changes as well. Our gated communities
of white segregation and concentrated advantage have to be opened
to low-income residents. Our communities of concentrated poverty
need concentrated reinvestment. This will require a redistribution of
wealth through taxation from the affluent back to the poor in the form
of living wages, access to higher education, free health care, and safe
housing. Only then will we cease to be a nation increasingly divided
by income and life expectancy. Inequality is a choice, not a random,
unfortunate set of circumstances. We can fix it, if we have the political
and economic nerve to do what's right.

THE THREE *B*s
BELIEFS, BEHAVIOR, BIOLOGY

Biological explanations have historically been a powerful way of convincing people that social inequality is natural and, therefore, does not require social change.... The biological explanation for inequality deludes people into thinking... that it's natural for black infants to die at two or three times the rate of white infants; it's natural for black people to be incarcerated at many times the rate of white people; it's natural for black children to have lower graduation rates than white children; it's natural for black people to have a fraction of the wealth white people have. Americans who don't want to explain these glaring inequities as stemming from institutionalized racism find comfort in explaining them as stemming from a natural order of human beings.[1]

DOROTHY ROBERTS

"I hear you are writing a book," the bejeweled woman to my left whispered. "What's the subject?"

I was at a dinner party in a well-appointed early-twentieth-century apartment with crown moldings and large French windows that overlooked the white-capped, blue-green expanse of Lake Michigan.

"It's about inequality in the United States as a cause of premature death," I replied. This was always a conversation stopper.

Her eyebrow arched. Before she had a chance to change the subject, I stormed in. I told her about the horrifying death gaps in Chicago and across the United States. I told her that despite all the advances in living conditions and medical care in the United States over the past century, which lifted overall life expectancy, many neighborhoods have been left behind, mired in ill health, misery, and poverty. I told her about structural violence and about how the vast accumulation of wealth and privilege in some communities is the reason such extreme poverty and high death rates exist elsewhere.

I could tell she was not buying it.

"I see these people at the supermarket all the time with their shopping carts filled with junk food," she said. "Then they pay for this bad food with their food stamps. Isn't it more about the way these people live and the choices they make?"

I wasn't surprised by this. Disbelief and skepticism are the usual responses when I raise the issue of structural violence and the death gap. People immediately jump to the three Bs—beliefs, behaviors, and biology—as the reasons for the health and life expectancy differences. And you cannot blame them. After all, not a day goes by that the news doesn't blast a story about diet or exercise: how eating nuts or brisk walking can lengthen one's life; how the poor are lazy and don't take care of themselves. My dinner mate's assertion that individual lifestyle beliefs and bad habits drive health outcomes is difficult to refute.

But it is incorrect.

Poor people *do* smoke more, do drink more, do use drugs more, are more obese, have more hypertension, more diabetes, more low-birth weight babies, more advanced cancers, and earlier heart disease than middle-class people. The bottom line: poor people die earlier than the middle class. So it is easy to assume that this is solely a result of poor people's behaviors and genes. A simple exploration of the Internet reinforces this way of thinking. Google the terms "poverty, genes and health" and up pop millions of hits with one outlandish claim after another, too often under the guise of scholarly research. Take, for instance, the article that postulated that gaps in the African gene pool are responsible for the deficiencies in African economic development and life expectancy.[2] Or the headline in the *Sunday Scotsman* that screamed "DOOMED TO FAILURE BY POVERTY GENE."[3] Research from the Glasgow Centre for Population Health postulated that centuries of natural selection among poor Scottish communities doomed those with low life expectancies to pass these poverty genes on, condemning the next generation to grow old before its time. Similarly, a *Salt Lake City Tribune* headline pronounced, "Poor, Uninsured Women Prone to Late-Stage Breast Cancer."[4] If you google "blacks, genetics and disease," you get 13,200,000 hits with similar claims of genetic causes for just about every disease imaginable. If you believe the headlines, the verdict is in.

But the truth is just the opposite, and there is an extensive scientific literature that shows just that. Unfortunately, there is also a long history of science contributing to the problem. Too often the scientific and medical establishment, to its shame, has endorsed or shored up explanations for inequality that rely on ostensibly racial, ethnic, and biologic evidence.

The Idea of Biological Inferiority

The idea that people with black and brown skin are biologically inferior to white-skinned people dates back centuries to the European colonization of Africa, Asia, and the Americas. Beliefs about the biological inferiority of blacks became central to justifications for slavery and for later white-supremacist laws that made race intermixing, including marriage, illegal in many states until the 1960s. Racism has permeated all of American society, including the fields of medicine and science.

Without denying that all diseases have biological manifestations (they would not be diseases if they did not), it would be biologically and evolutionarily preposterous to attribute diseases as wide ranging as breast cancer, hypertension, diabetes, renal failure, and tuberculosis to the genes that program melanin deposition in the skin. Yet a prevailing notion of race in biomedical and social research has assumed that traits like skin color can be used to categorize people into meaningful genetic subgroups to better understand disease and death predisposition. In our racially stratified society, biologic definitions of race have served to justify the naturalization of the social order. Legions of scientists have aimed to plumb the biological and genetic differences between races in order to validate the racial hierarchy. This has led to a widespread acceptance of the idea that biological explanations have some validity.

From Tuskegee to Oprah

While we no longer believe in phrenology and other antiquated forms of medical quackery, it is sobering to realize that some of the vilest expressions of scientific racism were conducted in mid-twentieth-century America. Perhaps the best known is the Tuskegee Experiment of Untreated Syphilis in the Negro Male, which was conducted by the US Public Health Services beginning in 1932 and left hundreds of men and their family members untreated until a reporter broke the story in 1972. The study was designed to evaluate how untreated syphilis affected blacks compared to whites. Although the PHS touted the study's scientific merit, it was pure scientific racism in its design and its perpetuation. Enrollees were never informed of the purpose of the research, nor did they give formal consent. The men were offered free medical care as part of the study—that is, their vulnerability as low-income people who otherwise did not have access to care was exploited. After penicillin treatment for syphilis became readily available in 1947, the untreated men were never offered it. Many suffered and possibly passed the infection to family members. It was not until 1996 that President Bill Clinton apologized on behalf of the federal government.

Tuskegee is hardly the only example of scientific racism. During World War II, secret experiments were conducted on 60,000 US soldiers, one of which involved exposing black and Puerto Rican soldiers to poison gas to see if they might be more resistant than whites to its toxic effects.[5] The army was contemplating using poison gas on the Japanese and was searching for the "ideal chemical soldier." Under threat of dishonorable discharge or imprisonment, some minority soldiers were placed in wooden shacks and gassed. Others were gassed from airplanes.

As National Public Radio reported, Rollins Edwards was one of the soldiers locked into a wooden gas chamber: "It felt like you were on fire," he recalled decades later. "Guys started screaming and hollering and trying to break out. And then some of the guys fainted. And finally they opened the door and let us out, and the guys were just, they were in bad shape." None of the soldiers received medical follow-up or VA benefits for the suffering they experienced.

Scientific racism remains common in present-day research. For example, researchers have promoted a theory that slavery is the reason for the high rates of hypertension in American blacks—that is, the extreme physical deprivation of the Middle Passage meant that only those slaves who were more able to retain salt and fluids survived. These slaves later produced offspring prone to developing hypertension.[6] This hypothesis, which has been soundly discredited, was reported extensively in the newspapers, in magazines, on the *Oprah Winfrey Show*, and in review articles that appeared in medical journals and textbooks.[7]

The advent of genomic and precision medicine has ushered in a new era of scientific racism. The Human Genome Project has unequivocally determined that human beings are 99.9 percent genetically alike. Yet genomic researchers have plunged into examination of the 0.1 percent of the genome to confront the "treacherous issue" of genetic differences between the races.[8] The increasingly popular but misguided view is that a tiny percentage of genetic difference among human beings might explain racial differences in disease incidence and mortality.

Environmental Racism and the Tragedy of Flint

Environmental racism is another example of structural violence. Chicago has among the highest child asthma mortality rates in the United States.[9] Black and Puerto Rican children are disproportionally affected, leading some to postulate racial and genetic etiologies.[10] Yet one cause has been traced back to a coal-burning power plant on the city's southwest side that spewed airborne particulates that poisoned the lungs of children in nearby neighborhoods.[11] Most of the children in these neighborhoods are black or Latino. Pediatric asthma mortality in Chicago was not a race issue; it was a place issue. Given Chicago's history of imposed neighborhood segregation, the real culprits were the racism and poverty that trapped children in these toxic wards.

The Flint, Michigan, lead poisoning crisis of 2016 is another example of structural environmental violence with a racist twist.[12] Flint, a Rust Belt city of 100,000, has been a victim of two generations of job loss and factory closings. Once a high-employment auto plant town, it teetered on the edge of solvency until the recession of 2008 knocked it into bankruptcy. The state of Michigan appointed a manager to act as a czar over the town's affairs. Democratic self-rule was yanked away from the mostly black city.[13] Because Flint could not afford to pipe in clean water from Lake Huron, the manager decided that the city should draw its drinking water from the toxic Flint River. Residents soon complained about the foul-smelling and -tasting water. State officials' reassurances about the safety of the water were in fact lies. The water was toxic, and its corrosive interaction with lead pipes caused an epidemic of lead poisoning among Flint children. Lead can cause permanent brain damage, as well as learning and behavioral problems in children. Poverty, racism, and systematic neglect are the unambiguous structural causes for this potentially lifelong health damage. The callous administrative act of switching the water supply was an act of structural violence. And the Flint poisoning must not be viewed as an isolated incident: across the country black children are more likely than white children to be poisoned by lead at levels higher than found in Flint.[14]

"Precision Medicine"

Race infects our discourse about health in so many ways. The search is on for race-specific and person-specific treatments for disease that pharmaceutical companies can commercialize. Over $200 billion is spent annually on prescription drugs in the United States. Unlike other developed countries, where pharmaceutical costs to consumers are strictly regulated, in the United States profit maximization is all but unregulated. Rocketing up 12 percent a year, pharmaceutical costs are the fastest-growing part of America's engorged health bill.[15]

Pharmaceutical companies, in search of new profits, have exploited debunked racist ideas about racial differences as biologically determined. The approval by the FDA of the first race-specific pharmaceutical has ushered in a new era of scientific racism in the guise of "precision medicine." Before 1997 there were no patents for race-specific pharmaceuticals, but between 2001 and 2005 there were sixty-five. In 2005 the FDA approved a drug, Bi-Dil, containing two common drugs that relax the blood vessels, specifically for the treatment of heart failure. The drug combo was shown to save lives in a randomized clinical experiment that was conducted with a group of self-reported African Americans. Given the evidence for Bi-Dil's efficacy, the FDA should have approved the drug for use by all heart failure patients.[16] But instead the FDA was persuaded to make its first race-specific pharmaceutical release. Most pharmaceutical clinical trials have been completed with only white participants, and the drugs have been approved for all patients regardless of race. But for Bi-Dil that generalizability was for some reason not acceptable. To portray Bi-Dil as a solution to a racial gap in mortality implies that the heart failure gap stems from racial differences in disease and drug response, for which there is no evidence. To argue that it is an example of "precision medicine" is misleading as well. The drugs are not targeting genomic differences. And it will not suffice to say that because it was never studied in whites, it is "precision medicine" for blacks. Race was used as a proxy for biological differences that have never been shown to exist. Given this, the Bi-Dil decision stands as a modern-day example of scientific racism.

The larger concern from the Bi-Dil release is that the drive of Big Pharma (as critics call the pharmaceutical industry) to commercialize findings from the human genome will lead to further racialization of science on false pretenses. Focusing on race at a molecular level while discounting its impact at a societal level can serve only to deflect attention from the real work that needs to be done.[17] And in the meantime, the general public reads about these decisions and believes that blacks' health outcomes have a biological basis.

The Embodiment of Racism and Poverty

If racial differences in health are not caused by biologic and genetic differences, how are we to understand the role of race and biology in health disparities? The United States does not have a universal methodology of identifying socioeconomic status in its vital statistics, so race and ethnicity have become stand-ins for social status in large-scale epidemiologic and population health studies. Race is an imprecise measure, however, not least because it is derived from self-reporting on census or hospital records and therefore could be inaccurate.

A more compelling perspective is that race is a political and social (not a biological) category. Think about this way. It has been well established that one's position in the social hierarchy is a predictor of longevity. Longitudinal studies of British civil servants demonstrated that administrators at the top of the hierarchy lived on average ten years longer than the janitors and others at the bottom.[18] At each rung lower in the ranks, mortality rates increased. This was despite the fact that everyone had access to the British National Health Service. Yet no one believes that those janitors are more biologically or genetically predisposed to die of heart disease than the top administrators.

Contrast this to the United States. Here, for just about all the diseases tracked by the government, blacks have higher disease and mortality rates than whites, even when income is controlled for. Analyses of the reasons for these gaps quickly devolve into debates about biological and genetic differences rather than the social gradient. This focus on biological explanations deflects attention from the real structural causes and potential solutions for America's death gaps. In modern times, life expectancy has tracked along an income and social gradient, yet it is irrational to claim that the reason for the fifteen-year life-expectancy gap between the lowest-income 1 percent of Americans (a group that includes many black Americans) and the highest-income 1 percent is biological.[19]

To think about race as a political classification requires us to redirect our causal explanations for racial inequities from the biological to the political structures of governance and social control that drive the inequities. This requires a shift of perspective about diseases and their treatments. If diseases are just biological events occurring within a person, then they require treatments directed only at the individual. But if we believe that racism and poverty cause diseases and premature mortality, then the solutions have to be directed at the economic systems and political structures that are perpetuating them.

But all diseases have biological manifestations. So what are the mechanisms by which structural violence causes disease to manifest? Dr. Nancy Krieger, a professor at the Harvard School of Public Health who has studied racial health inequities, postulates that people biologically embody their life experiences in societal and ecologic contexts.[20]

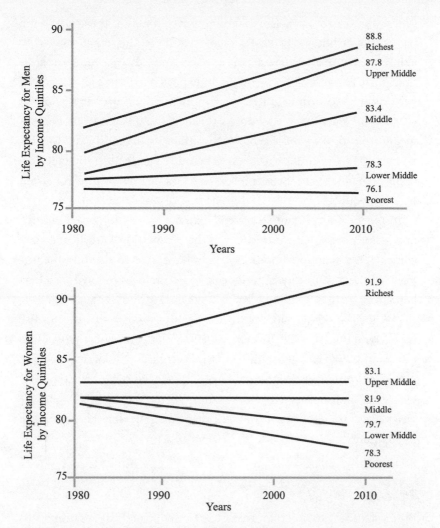

Life expectancy in the United States operates along an income gradient, but that gap has widened over time. Since 1980, those in the highest quintile of income (the richest) are seeing greater strides in life expectancy than those in the lowest two quintiles (lower middle and poorest). For those two groups, life expectancies have remained flat or have decreased. Source: Committee Generated from Health and Retirement Study Data.

This embodiment of racism and poverty accounts for the some of the patterns of health and disease we see. Health inequity is shaped not by a simple relationship between an exposure and a disease but by a series of exposures over a lifetime or, when experienced intra-utero, across generations. According to Krieger, the greater the power and resource inequality in a society, the more prevalent the disease outcome, the greater the absolute disease burden on those with less power. Racism and other forms of discrimination therefore can lead to the embodiment of inequality in the form of disease and lead to population-wide health inequities.

In recent years, scientists have been measuring "perceived racism" and linking personal experiences of discrimination with health outcomes. More than one hundred studies have tried to measure the impacts of the day-to-day experiences nonwhite people have—such as being followed in a store by a clerk or being stopped or harassed by the police—and correlate them with health outcomes. These studies have found that people who experienced high degrees of personal discrimination had worse health outcomes across a series of diseases. For example, women who had experienced high levels of perceived racism over their lifetimes were five times more likely to deliver a low-birthweight baby than those who did not.[21] This suggests that the experience of inequality causes disease.

Poverty, Race, or Both?

But biological explanations are not the only flawed explanations that people believe. There are many who say that the black-to-white death gap in the United States is not a product of racism but exclusively a product of education, poverty, and income inequality. This is also wrong, as it ignores structural racism as a unique and powerful transmitter of violence.

We have known for decades that better-educated, richer people live longer than poorer, less-educated people. In 1980, people with family incomes in the top 5 percent had life expectancies about 25 percent higher than those in the bottom 5 percent.[22] We also know that compared to whites, blacks have less education and lower income, so poverty itself is a driver of black-to-white health inequality.

Yet a growing global literature posits that it is not poverty alone but the overall income inequality in a society that drives life expectancy rates down. The studies, while not conclusive, have posited that the greater the income inequality, the greater the hazard to the health of a society.[23] Angus Deaton, a Nobel Prize–winning Princeton professor of economics, analyzed income inequality and mortality across the United States.[24] He found at both the state and metropolitan levels that mortality is positively correlated with almost any measure of income inequality, both in the aggregate and for black and white mortality separately. He also found that income inequality and mortality rates are higher in areas with more blacks. When controlled for the proportion of black people, the effect of income inequality disappeared. What really seems to matter, according to Deaton, when it comes to mortality inequality in the United States, is the fraction of blacks in a city or state: the more black people, the higher the death rate. How can this be? From a public health perspective, it is epidemiologically impossible to tease out the separate contributions of racism and poverty to the death gaps in America. Suffice it to say that the preponderance of the evidence suggests that both racism and poverty perpetuated by loosely regulated free-market capitalism are structural forces that contribute to premature mortality in synergistic ways.

Centuries of scientific racism have allowed focus to be deflected from the structural to behavioral and biological causes of health inequality. Deaton notes that if poverty is the result of "poor institutions, poor government and toxic politics," then the cure needs to be aimed at those institutions.[25] The same is true of health inequities. A renewed attention on the structural cures for racism and poverty in America's abandoned neighborhoods would reverse health inequities and reduce death gaps.

The good news in this sad amalgamation of data is that we have the means to reverse these mortality trends. There are individuals and communities that have been able to resist and overcome aspects of structural violence.[26] Being poor can be deadly, but it is not as deadly in every neighborhood or every region of the country.[27] We can learn from these local and regional differences. Structural violence can be mitigated. But not before we start to better understand our biases and how hardwired these racist notions of disease causality have become.

Conversation Over

Back at my dinner party, I leaned in toward my companion to explain some of this. "Individual health behaviors are often swamped by large-scale social and structural phenomena such as poverty, joblessness, discrimination, lack of health insurance and education as causes of premature death. Poverty, racism, and other forms of structural violence are thieves. They sap the life from individuals who live in disadvantaged communities. Individual risk factors and unhealthy behaviors are just a small part of the story. Taken all in, the preponderance of poor health outcomes in these neighborhoods is not the result of bad choices, bad luck, or bad biology. Rather it was born of deliberate economic and public policies that dictate neighborhood education, housing, food, health care choices, and mobility. These policies favor the top 20 percent and target the poor and minorities with deadly consequences."

I know that I need to tone it down for certain audiences. My dinner mate had thought she was coming to a fancy party for great food and "witty repartee," not a lecture from some guy channeling the Occupy and Black Lives Matter movements. Her eyes narrowed as she served me a polite mother-of-pearl smile that announced, "Conversation over."

I need to get better at making the case to folks like her, for the sake of people like Windora Bradley and her family.

Neighborhoods, Stress, and Premature Illness

There is a way in which neighborhoods, biology, and longevity are intertwined, but it has to do with stress, not racial difference. People who are exposed to constant high levels of stress do have biological reactions that can shorten their lives. Conversely, removing people from these stressful situations can improve their health.

Take the case of Cora Murphy, Windora Bradley's sister, who used to live upstairs from her in Humboldt Park. Both were overweight. Both had diabetes and hypertension. Then one day Cora met a computer technician at the junior high school where she managed the cafeteria. Mr. Murphy was in his late sixties and a former Black Panther who had helped run the free children's breakfast program the Panthers established in the 1970s in Chicago—a precursor to public school–based food programs. But he had eventually moved out of the city to the grassy south suburbs. Cora married Murphy and moved from her inner-city neighborhood to his suburban home. She and I discussed the changes to her health about six months after she moved.

She told me she had begun to exercise every day. I checked her Hemoglobin A1C, a measure of diabetes control, and found that her diabetes and blood pressure were better managed. In fact, her diabetes was in the best control it had been for years. When I told her this, she smiled.

This is one story from one patient, but Cora's anecdotal experience reaffirms the notion that certain neighborhoods are bad for health while others are better. The scientific research on the biological effects of concentrated poverty and disadvantage is recent and compelling. A growing set of discoveries suggests that exposure to chronic environmental stress causes biological changes within the body that predispose individuals to develop premature disease.[28] High ambient and psychosocial stress activates the neuroendocrine system in the body, the "fight or flight" mechanism. Stress-triggered stimulant substances, such as epinephrine, whoosh into the blood from the adrenal glands, raising heart rate and blood pressure. Then in a cascade of events, the "stress hormone" cortisol and other activated inflammatory promoting factors are released from cells.[29]

These are ancient and important defense mechanisms, the same that kept our ancestors from the clutches of saber-toothed tigers and other predators. But frequent cycles of stress like those in impoverished neighborhoods challenge the body's ability to remain in homeostasis or steady state.[30] The impact of repeated cycles of stress and hormone activation is called the "allostatic load," and stress-induced shifts in allostatic load can permanently raise blood pressure, induce plaque formation in arteries, and cause organ failure.[31] Diseases such as metabolic syndrome (the triad of central obesity, glucose intolerance, and hypertension) are believed to have their roots in these cycles.[32] Stress-induced high cortisol levels stimulate appetite through a number of mechanisms including the release of ghrelin, a peptide that stimulates hunger. However, ghrelin released during chronic stress also makes the brain more susceptible to posttraumatic stress disorder (PTSD).[33] Therefore, repeated allostatic insults may lead to obesity with its attendant consequences: diabetes, hypertension, premature heart disease, and PTSD.[34]

In addition to allostatic load, midlife adults and the elderly living in disadvantaged inner-city neighborhoods exhibit higher levels of pro-inflammatory factors in their blood than those living in advantaged neighborhoods.[35] These factors are known to predispose individuals to premature heart disease.[36] While much of this evidence is circumstantial, it does give credence to the idea that chronic stress and the biologic changes it causes predispose individuals to premature disease and death. Windora Bradley was a textbook example of this.

Stress during Pregnancy

But is it true that these stresses and their impacts can be passed from generation to generation as Krieger suggests? Many studies have investigated the effects of stress during pregnancy on offspring. Animal studies are quite definitive that stress in utero leads to premature birth and low birth weight.[37] This is one way in which mortality risks can be transmitted from one generation to another. In humans, mothers who report high levels of stress are also more likely to have low-birth-weight babies.[38] In turn, these babies are more susceptible to hypertension later in life.[39] In the United States, black women have the highest percentage of low-birth-weight babies of any race or ethnic group,[40] but babies born to African women do not have the same degree of low birth weight, which gives more credence to the idea that racism and placeism are the culprits, not bad genes.[41] That black women who report having experienced specific discriminatory behaviors have lower-birthweight babies than those who do not have those experiences also supports the intergenerational transmission of structural violence.[42]

Biological Weathering

A more recent inquiry has looked at the effect of stress on aging. Nobel Prize–winning biologist Elizabeth Blackburn has studied the effect of stress on telomere length.[43] Telomeres are the active tips of chromosomes that are found in just about every cell in the body. These tiny repeat sequences of DNA protect the cell's genetic stability by "capping" the ends of chromosomes to prevent degeneration. When exposed to chronic stress, telomeres are shortened; the shorter the telomere, the older the biological age.[44] This stress-induced shortening has been termed "biological weathering." Scientists postulate that black women in the United States experience more weathering than other groups due to a chronic overload of environmental stressors. Based on telomere analysis, black women in the United States between the ages of 49 and 55 are 7.5 years older biologically due to this weathering effect, with perceived stress and poverty accounting for almost 30 percent of the age gap.[45] So in short, social inequality causes stress, leading to shortened telomeres and, in turn, premature aging, disease, and early death.[46]

A Tale of Two Cities

What can be done to break these vicious cycles? Is it enough for people to move, as Cora did, from a high-stress community of concentrated disadvantage to a community of concentrated advantage? In lower-stress and lower-poverty environments, does health really improve? While it is difficult to run controlled trials on neighborhood effects on health, there is some evidence that moving to a better neighborhood does have lasting health benefits. (I will discuss this further in chapter 10.)

What is clear is that a person's zip code can be more influential than his or her genetic code. We can see the zip-code effect with startling clarity if we consider black infant mortality in two Wisconsin counties. In Racine County, the gap in the mortality rate between black and white infants was among the highest in the nation in 2008.[47] But one hundred miles west in Dane County, between 2004 and 2007 the gap was nonexistent.[48] Ta-Shai Pendleton's story suggests an explanation. Her first and second pregnancies were problematic—one stillborn, one premature. Both births occurred in Racine County. Not until she moved from Racine to Madison did she successfully give birth following a full-term pregnancy. Public health experts were at a loss to name a single factor that was responsible for the drop in black infant mortality in Madison. Instead they ascribed the improvements to a community effect. According to the county health director, "Pregnant women need to feel safe, cared for and valued.... When they don't, that contributes to premature birth and fetal loss in the six or seventh month." Madison is filled with better and more varied public and private services than those available in Racine County. It is less segregated and less violent and has less poverty with more accessible heath care and community support than the cities of Racine and Milwaukee.[49] And while the infant mortality gap has reappeared in Dane County since the 2008 recession, preterm infant births among blacks have continued to remain lower than the national rate.[50]

Cora's and Ta-Shai's mobility from high- to low-poverty neighborhoods is the exception among the poor in the United States. Many impoverished Americans are stuck in place—sometimes over generations, and thus they are subject to the chronic, relentless, and deleterious effects of place on health.[51]

Changing the Opinions of Skeptics

I cannot blame my dinner mate for her views about the effects of beliefs, behaviors, and biology on our physical and mental well-being. Our ideas on race, poverty, and health in the United States are tempered by strongly held social beliefs and cultural norms that posit personal responsibility as a core factor in achieving good health. My job as a doctor is to encourage patients like Cora to exercise more, to change their diet, and otherwise to choose a healthy lifestyle. I would be the last to claim that individual responsibility for health is unimportant.

Risk-factor reduction has been responsible for a portion of overall improvements in life expectancy over the last century. But as a social epidemiologist I know these words of encouragement and counseling will have little impact on the overall death gaps in the United States unless we address structural violence and the triple evils of poverty, placeism, and racism.

PART 2
TRAPPED BY INEQUITY

6

FIRE AND RAIN

LIFE AND DEATH IN NATURAL DISASTERS

Medical statistics will be our standard of measurement: we will weigh life for life and see where the dead lie thicker, among the workers or among the privileged.[1]

RUDOLF VIRCHOW (1848)

It Takes a Disaster

If you are an affluent white man in the United States, you may never have to witness the human impact of structural violence. Our highways tend to bypass high-mortality neighborhoods. If we find ourselves in a high-poverty area, we lock the doors, roll the windows up, and accelerate. If you do not live or work in a high-poverty neighborhood, you have likely never witnessed the suffering up close. The people who live there are not your friends, coworkers, or family members. The violence inflicted on the residents of these forgotten neighborhoods is out of sight and out of mind. Our towns and communities can seem hermetically sealed off from these invisible distressed neighborhoods, though they're often just a short drive away. Our grocery stores, our schools, our shopping areas, and our hospitals are separate and sedate. Structural violence is only an intellectual notion to be debated or ignored. Why would we want to interrupt the comfort of our lives to address the nature and distribution of the extreme suffering beyond our neighborhoods?

But sometimes all Americans become spectators of the death and destruction wreaked by violence. When a natural disaster hits, the media spotlight often turns to America's impoverished neighborhoods. Anderson Cooper arrives with cameras rolling. Disaster-preparedness crews are deployed. The sirens and red and orange strobe lights of emergency vehicles pierce the night. Public officials in tieless shirts, baseball caps, and bombardier jackets walk around shaking hands and looking concerned. For a brief moment, the whole world is watching. Invisible truths about America's hidden human disaster zones become visible during these moments of natural calamity.

We think of extreme weather events as "acts of God," indiscriminate in the death and destruction they cause. But this is not the case. The Chicago heat wave of 1995 and the aftermath of Hurricane Katrina in New Orleans in 2005 were environmental disasters that exposed structural flaws in American society. Both exposed the social fault lines of poverty, geography, and race. In both cities, the most fragile neighborhoods had been in disaster states for years: high poverty, limited mobility, substandard housing, high illness and mortality rates. Social networks had been frayed by mass imprisonment and joblessness. In both cities, emergency management plans failed to account for the fragility and special needs of the residents of these chronically distressed neighborhoods, and many lives were lost as a result. Worst of all, whatever lessons were learned in Chicago in 1995 were not applied in New Orleans in 2005.

In both cities, as bodies piled up and officials struggled to wrestle with the unfolding human disaster, the narrative was deflected away from the inadequacy of the emergency planning and response. The victims and their communities were blamed for the suffering and death that ensued. This was structural violence at its most obscene and most appalling.

Tropical Chicago

As the Chicago Cubs faced the Cincinnati Reds at Wrigley Field on Thursday, July 13, 1995, people were suffering in record numbers across the city. A treacherous hot, high-pressure air mass had slid into Chicago in early July and stalled there, causing record-high temperatures. Chicago gets hot in the summer, but that week the weather was like that in Bombay.

Cars overheated and stalled. Roads buckled. Rail tracks warped. Chicago River drawbridges had to be hosed down so they could close. As game time approached, the temperature was 106 degrees Fahrenheit and the heat index was 125, the highest on record. So many air conditioners were cranked full throttle that Commonwealth Edison instituted rolling blackouts to manage the demand, crippling neighborhoods. Emergency rooms swarmed with patients suffering from heat stroke and dehydration. The 911 call center was besieged with distress calls and could not keep pace. Paramedics crisscrossed the city to yank victims from overheated homes, but twenty of the city's hospitals, those serving the poorest communities in Chicago, had become so overcrowded that they instructed ambulances to avoid them.

The sweating vendors at Wrigley Field had a record night selling beer and Pepsi to the roasting fans. The starting pitcher that night for the Cubs was Steve Trachsel, nicknamed "the Human Rain Delay" because of his slothlike pace. That night he seemed even more deliberate than usual—at least until he got yanked in the second inning. I was at Wrigley that night with Dr. Steve Whitman, then the director of epidemiology for the Chicago Department of Health. While we sweltered in the box seats and downed Pepsi after Pepsi, the Chicago Heat Wave was on its way to killing more than seven hundred Chicagoans, mostly residents of neighborhoods of concentrated poverty. Little did we know that Whitman was to play the leading role in our subsequent understanding of this epidemic. His sleuthing helped uncover the structural violence at the root of the heat wave deaths.

Corpses Accumulate, Mayor Vacations

Ed Donahue, Cook County's medical examiner, had the ghoulish job of determining the cause of death for corpses that were brought to his offices on any given day. Usually there were about a dozen of them, mostly people who had died of natural causes. On hot summer nights, some of them were young victims of urban trauma. Sometimes an examiner would call me about a patient of mine who had died at home. I would provide the relevant background information, and the examiner would assign a cause of death where it was unclear. Donahue's office had a rule of thumb. If you were older than forty-five and you died without evidence of foul play, you likely died of cardiovascular disease. It was rare for the office to perform an autopsy on anyone suspected of dying from cardiovascular disease.

But between July 14 and July 20, the ambulances deposited body after body, so many that there was nowhere to store them. A local meat-packing firm lent a 48-foot refrigerated truck. Then it sent another, and another, and another until there were nine of them in the morgue's parking lot.

Donahue and his staff scrambled to understand what was happening. The stories were all similar. The fire department was called to an overheated apartment. They found a corpse, generally of an older person who had lived alone. A 79-year-old black man found dead on Wednesday, July 19, was typical of the victims. The records kept by the responding police officers noted: "Victim did not respond to calls or knocks on victim's door since Sunday.... Victim was known as quiet, [kept] to himself.... Chain was on door.... Victim on sofa with flies on victim and a very strong odor of decay."[2]

Donahue began to label these heat-related deaths, instead of deaths from cardiovascular disease. The classic and most conservative definition of heat-related mortality (whether heat stroke, heat exhaustion, or hyperthermia) relied on measuring core body temperatures at or near the time of death. In this week, Donahue based his designation not only on body temperatures but also on the mere fact that the death had occurred during the heat wave, with no other obvious cause. An autopsy on a victim of heat stroke would look no different from one on someone who died of cardiovascular collapse. It was the environmental conditions that allowed Donahue to call these deaths heat related.

As the bodies piled up, the Chicago press corps began to take notice. Donahue, always a straight talker, told them the deaths were a citywide tragedy: "This continues to be a disaster, Never before in the city of Chicago could anyone have predicted this kind of a problem."[3]

The city government faced intense criticism. The city had not de-

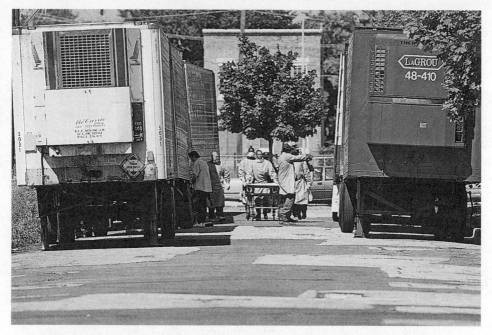

Unclaimed bodies, victims of the 1995 Chicago Heat Wave, were kept in these massive refrigerated trucks before being moved to mass graves. There were 739 deaths, many preventable, making this the biggest single human disaster in Chicago's history, with more than twice as many deaths as those in the Chicago Fire of 1871. Source: AP Images.

clared an environmental emergency. Chicago had not established emergency cooling centers. It had not organized door-to-door checks in high-risk neighborhoods. Officials had not handed out fans or air conditioners. In fact, Mayor Richard M. Daley and other city officials were out of town. As the heat approached, they had escaped to their Michigan summer homes. Then, while the corpses accumulated, they delayed their returns.

More affluent Chicagoans had the ability to cool their homes with air conditioning. Those with second homes could flee the city. But thousands of old, poor, isolated, and sick Chicagoans, especially those in black neighborhoods, had no relief from the lethal conditions. City tenements with black tar roofs on treeless streets baked like ovens. Most of those who died had poorly functioning air conditioners, or none. Others died after sleeping inside with closed windows, some of which were nailed shut for fear of crime. In those cases, one form of structural violence was abetting another.

A War of Water and Words

In many of these roasting neighborhoods, the police cracked down on teens who opened over fire hydrants to cool off—more than seven hundred were opened. Images of "water wars" featured prominently in the local media. Meanwhile in a war of words, city officials protested that all precautions had been taken. Human Services commissioner Daniel Alvarez criticized the victims. "We are talking about people who die because they neglect themselves," he said. "We did everything possible. But some people didn't want to even open their doors to us."[4]

Mayor Daley, back in town and ever sensitive to criticism, began to take umbrage at Donahue's claim that 550 deaths—mostly isolated elderly, sick people from poor neighborhoods—were heat related. Daley insisted that the deaths were from natural causes: these were frail elderly people who were likely to die soon anyway. Said Daley on July 17: "It's hot. It's very hot. We all have our little problems but let's not blow it out of proportion.... We go to extremes in Chicago. And that's why people like Chicago. We go to extremes."

"Every day people die of natural causes," Daley said at a news conference the next day. "You cannot claim that everybody who has died in the last eight or nine days dies of heat. Then everybody in the summer that dies will die of heat."[5]

I Am Only a Mathematician

Steve Whitman followed the clash between the mayor and the medical examiner. He knew that with some sleuthing he could pinpoint how many people had died and what neighborhoods were hit hardest. As a social epidemiologist, he was particularly interested in the role neighborhoods and conditions such as racism and poverty had on disease incidence and mortality. He explained his particular take on disease and its causes in an interview in 2012:

Epidemiology is considered thinking about the distribution of disease in populations; and social epidemiology just means doing that, paying attention to social factors like racism and poverty and their correlates. For example: lack of food, poor schools, violence, having a place to exercise in the community, and things of that sort.... You just don't look at what proportion of people has diabetes, but you try to understand, say, the difference between different groups and how that in turn is a function of racism and poverty.[6]

As Whitman investigated the Chicago Heat Wave, he first sought to determine how many of the deaths between July 14 and July 20 could be considered excess deaths. On average, about seventy-two Chicagoans died every day. If, as Mayor Daley declared, the people who died in the heat wave died of natural causes a little sooner than expected, the spike in deaths during the heat wave should be followed by a large drop in deaths afterward, so that over time the average remained the same.

There certainly was a big spike in deaths corresponding with the peak of the heat wave. Whitman calculated that on Saturday, July 15, two days after the hottest day to date in Chicago, 275 more people died than expected. There *was* a dip in post–heat wave deaths, but it was far overshadowed by the tidal wave of premature mortality. As Donahue has said, the excess deaths were likely due to the heat itself. But the number of excess deaths Whitman calculated was more than 30 percent higher than the 550 that Donahue had counted: 739. In the early days of the heat wave, the medical examiner might not have ascribed all the deaths to the heat wave, or he might not have had accurate temperature readings from the sites where the bodies were found.

Word of Whitman's calculation percolated through the health department to City Hall. If true, it was one of the worst human disasters in Chicago's history. It was a major embarrassment to the mayor and the city officials, who had been in a state of denial about the emergency. Whitman was summoned to the mayor's office. He was ushered into a wood-paneled conference room. The doors were locked behind him. Stone-faced aides and city attorneys demanded that conversations at the meeting remain secret. The mayor had been so vociferous in denying that the heat was causing deaths that they had a political problem on their hands if their own health department proclaimed 739 deaths.

"How can you say they are heat-related deaths?" the lawyers protested. "They are only numbers!"

"I am only a mathematician," Whitman responded, tongue in cheek. They were only numbers, but they depicted a callous and unprepared city administration. And Whitman's analysis did not stop there.

Whitman's data revealed a darker side of the mortality from the heat wave.[7] Decades of structural violence were responsible for the high death rates. Not all neighborhoods or all people were targeted equally. Older, socially isolated people died at a higher rate than younger people. Black people were almost 50 percent more likely to die during the heat wave than white people. Eight of the ten neighborhoods with the highest heat wave mortality were black neighborhoods of concentrated poverty. One of the hardest-hit black neighborhoods was North Lawndale, devastated for twenty-five years or more by structural forces like blockbusting, loss of jobs and housing, and high rates of homicide, infant mortality, and deaths from breast cancer and cardiovascular conditions. Whitman's analysis reinforced the fact that place and race matter as much as personal characteristics in predicting death.

Some neighborhoods were more resilient than others during the heat wave. Englewood and Auburn Gresham are contiguous black neighborhoods with concentrated poverty and crime. But the death rate in Englewood during the heat wave was thirty times that in Auburn Gresham. South Lawndale is a Mexican community adjacent to North Lawndale and is a high-poverty area. Yet South Lawndale's death rate was among the lowest in Chicago—one-tenth the rate of North Lawndale. South Lawndale is a community of immigrants from Mexico; it's possible that the elderly there face less social isolation than people in North Lawndale do.

An analysis of the root cause of the deaths identified a number of interventions that could have saved lives. More than half the lives might have been saved if the victims had had air conditioning, either in their homes or in shelters. Other lives could have been saved had the city initiated its emergency preparedness plan earlier or asked for help from other political jurisdictions. Meteorologists had at least one week's warning that severe weather was approaching Chicago, so there was ample time to plan. This did not happen. The 739 deaths made the Chicago Heat Wave one of America's worst environmental disasters ever, surpassing the death toll from the 1871 Chicago Fire and the San Francisco Earthquake of 1906.

Black, Poor, and Left Behind

Ten years later, as Category Five Hurricane Katrina with 120-mile-per-hour winds bore down on New Orleans, it seemed as if all the lessons from the Chicago Heat Wave had been forgotten or ignored by the federal government, the State of Louisiana, and the City of New Orleans. Nothing could have been done to blunt the fury of the storm. But natural disasters have a way of exposing the crevices in society, and the images from New Orleans in the aftermath of the hurricane and the breached levees revealed a social tragedy similar to that revealed by the Chicago Heat Wave. And as in Chicago, the tragedy in New Orleans was as predictable as it was preventable.

Katrina provided another horrific example of what can happen when environmental forces intersect with a social geography resulting from years of social neglect, racism, and urban decay. Over the previous century, as low-lying wetlands were drained to accommodate a growing population in New Orleans, a new social geography had been created based on race and poverty. Decades of white flight from New Orleans to suburban areas left vast regions of concentrated black poverty, many located in areas below sea level. The neighborhoods on higher ground were more likely to be white ones. The most vulnerable of the city's black neighborhoods were among the most impoverished in the United States. Of the almost 30 percent of New Orleans residents living below the poverty level before Katrina, 84 percent were black.[8]

The widespread destructive force of Katrina affected people of all races and economic means across the Gulf Coast. Many suffered. Livelihoods were destroyed. But when the order to evacuate was given, the most vulnerable did not have the means to do so. Many had never been beyond the city limits and had nowhere to go. Others were too frail or ill to move. At least 25 percent of the New Orleans population did not have a car.[9] Katrina's arrival simply exposed decades of social inequity with its entrenched historical roots.

A Fatally Flawed Plan

The emergency management plan in New Orleans was fatally flawed. It called for those without automobiles to be helped by those who did (this was termed the "Good Samaritan plan") or urged survivors to seek shelter in the Superdome. What followed was as horrifying as it was predictable.

Those who remained in New Orleans after the mandatory evacuation order were largely black, elderly, sick, and poor residents of inner-city lowland areas. More than 20,000 of them did seek refuge at the Superdome, which became a place of squalor and desperation, with inadequate food and sanitary supplies. Dead bodies were lined up on the loading dock. One corpse sat in a folding chair outside the Superdome's entrance. Buses to evacuate the population were delayed for days. People needing help, victims of an incompetent emergency response, began to be viewed as threats to the social order, as false or exaggerated reports spread of shooting, looting, raping, and more inside the Superdome.

Despite the lack of preparation on the local, state, and federal levels, after the disaster hit national officials blamed those who failed to evacuate as "getting what they deserved." In response to rising death tolls, Federal Emergency Management Agency director Michael Brown told Congress, "That's going to be attributable a lot to people… who chose not to leave."[10] Structural violence had claimed another victim: basic human empathy.

Those who evacuated before the storm hit were mostly white and mostly middle class. Those who stayed were mostly black and mostly working class. Those who fled before the storm had privileges that most middle-class Americans take for granted: education, money, reliable access to transportation, social networks that extended farther away from the hurricane-hit area, and access to news reports to warn them of the storm's severity. Those left behind had none of these advantages.[11]

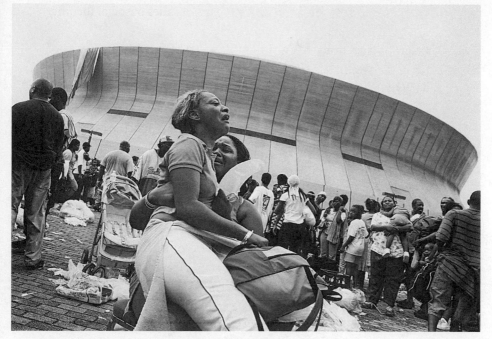

New Orleans residents congregate at the Superdome after Hurricane Katrina. Source: *New York Daily News* Archive.

Debbie Este was one of these victims. Wheelchair bound and living in a small house with her 68-year-old disabled mother and two teenage daughters, she watched her mother die of heart failure as the flood-waters rose and forced them to their attic. They sweltered without food or water next to the lifeless body of Debbie's mother. Their screams for help went unanswered for three days. Debbie felt so hopeless that she suggested to her daughters that they end their lives by overdosing on her painkillers: "I said no one is going to save us here and I don't want to die like this, three days laying in this stinky, dirty water."

Debbie and her daughters made it out alive but were representative of the dilemma facing the poor and vulnerable inhabitants of New Or-leans. Survival came with a price. They witnessed the death of a loved one. They contemplated suicide. They were displaced. And then they were blamed for what happened to them. The impact of this disaster would linger in their lives long after the waters receded.[12]

Blame Game

The news images from New Orleans perpetuated the stereotype of poor black people as threats to public order. The imagery of black poverty and destitution on the nightly news shocked Americans for whom the reality of this extreme inequality was invisible in daily life. These stories deflected attention from the flagrant incompetence of the rescue mission to the victims of the hurricane. The Associated Press on August 30 showed an image of a black man wading through chest-deep water with food that he had "looted" from a grocery store. On the same day, the AFP/Getty press agency showed a picture of a white couple wading through similar water after "finding" food at a grocery store. By framing blacks as looters and whites as survivors, the media perpetuated the idea that blacks are criminals and social deviants. There was little coverage given to the way that extended black families and others supported themselves through this crisis when government relief efforts failed.

Similarly, the media described the whites who escaped New Orleans by car and airplane in the days preceding the hurricane as "evacuees," while the mostly black and poor residents trapped behind were called "refugees." Many in the African American community protested the use of this term as further evidence of the depictions of black poverty in the United States as otherworldly, pathological, and un-American. Tyrone McKnight resisted the depiction as he sat outside a Baton Rouge shelter where he had been evacuated with thousands of other New Orleans residents: "The image I have in my mind is people in a Third World country, the babies in Africa that have all the flies and are starving to death. That's not me. I'm a law-abiding citizen who's working every day and paying taxes."[13]

Katrina's Health Consequences

Beyond the reinforcing of stereotypes, there were substantial health consequences of Katrina, and perhaps by now it is no surprise that black and poor people were disproportionally affected. Fifty-one percent

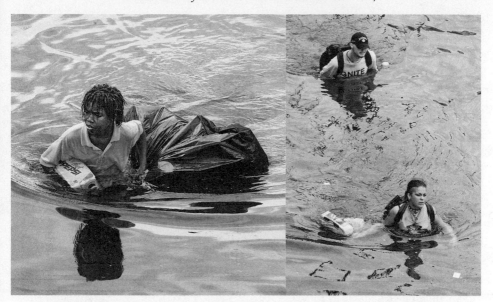

The Associated Press on August 30, 2005, showed an image of a black man wading through chest-deep water with food that he had "looted" from a grocery store. On the same day, the AFP/Getty press agency showed a picture of a white couple wading through similar water after "finding" food at a grocery store. By framing blacks as looters and whites as survivors, the media perpetuated the idea that blacks are criminals and social deviants. Sources: photographer Chris Graythen and photographer Dave Martin, AP.

of the nearly 2,000 New Orleans Katrina deaths were black people.[14] The three most common causes of death were drowning, trauma, and heart disease. Blacks in New Orleans died 1.7 to 4 times more often than whites. Four out of five communities with the highest death rates were black neighborhoods. The community with the highest death rate was the Lower Ninth Ward, which suffered extensive flooding from the levee breaches. As in the Chicago Heat Wave, the elderly experienced a higher death rate than those under 75, and neighborhoods with higher chronic-disease death gaps before the storm were also the ones that saw high disaster-related mortality rates. Post-Katrina, rates of mental disorders like depression, PTSD, and mold-related respiratory diseases rose, again disproportionately affecting poor black people.

Structural Violence and Preventable Death

The disproportionate deaths in the black communities in both the Chicago Heat Wave and Katrina were manifestations of structural violence. In both environmental disasters, members of communities of concentrated disadvantage died because of the failures of the political, emergency response, and public health structures—structures that had been failing black neighborhoods for years. In both cities, insufficient emergency management plans put the population at risk and caused many preventable deaths. In New Orleans, the breach of the levee that flooded low-lying black neighborhoods had been predicted, but repairs that could have mitigated the flooding were not funded in time. In the ten years after Katrina, only 37 percent of the homes in the Lower Ninth Ward were rebuilt, compared to 90 percent of homes elsewhere in New Orleans. In Chicago, city residents fared better during the heat wave of 2012 because of an emergency plan that now includes cooling centers, air conditioners, and door-to-door checks on the frail. While emergency management plans in both cities have improved in the aftermaths, the neighborhood conditions that spawned the high death rates have not. Both natural disasters forced the nation to witness, for a brief moment, the ongoing disaster of concentrated poverty and squalor of inner-city black neighborhoods. But neither disaster led to the kind of community reinvestment necessary to relieve suffering and bring fundamental change to these neighborhoods.

MASS INCARCERATION, PREMATURE DEATH, AND COMMUNITY HEALTH

In the era of colorblindness, it is no longer socially permissible to use race, explicitly, as a justification for discrimination, exclusion, and social contempt. So we don't. Rather than rely on race, we use our criminal justice system to label people of color "criminals" and then engage in all the practices we supposedly left behind. Today it is perfectly legal to discriminate against criminals in nearly all the ways that it was once legal to discriminate against African Americans.... We have not ended racial caste in America; we have merely redesigned it.[1]

MICHELLE ALEXANDER

To improve life expectancy in America, we must improve the living conditions for people in our most distressed neighborhoods. To improve living conditions for people in our most distressed neighborhoods, we must combat structural violence. To combat structural violence, we must battle the dual evils of racism and poverty. To battle the dual evils of racism and poverty, we must end mass incarceration, as it is one driver of poor health and poverty. There are other remedies required to improve community health outcomes, too, but if we are serious about improving life expectancy, mass incarceration—a uniquely American system of racial and social control—has to be stopped. Mass incarceration is a public health epidemic. Its impact is huge for those held captive in the system but also devastating for the overall health of disadvantaged communities.

1.5 Million Missing Black Men

In the 1960s and 1970s, black Americans gained the full rights of citizenship that had been denied to them for centuries. As they won the right to vote, move freely, ride public transportation, and attend public school, the United States constructed an unprecedented penal system, calculated, some believe, to reverse the gains achieved by the civil rights movement.[2] Today the impact of the mass imprisonment can be felt in almost every black neighborhood in America. The problem is most acute in urban black communities. Take Chicago: the incarceration rate in the best black community there is forty times higher than the incarceration rate in the best white neighborhood.[3]

In neighborhoods across the nation, middle-aged black men are absent. In most white neighborhoods the ratio of men to women is about equal. For every 100 white women in the prime of their lives, there are 99 white men. But across America, for every 100 black women ages 24 to 54, there are only 83 black men. The others—one of every six—are missing. If you add up all the missing black men, it is a staggering number: 1.5 million nationwide.[4]

Where have these men gone? Almost 900,000 of them are prematurely dead. While homicide, from the epidemic of urban gun violence, is responsible for a portion of these premature deaths, most of them are from heart disease and cancer. About 600,000 24- to 54-year-old men are in prison at any given time, a condition that also shortens their lifespans. Prison has medical consequences, just like any disease.

Black men are missing from communities large and small. In Ferguson, Missouri, there are only 60 men, ages 25 to 54, for every 100 women of the same ages. In New York City there are 118,000 missing black men between the ages of 25 and 54. In Chicago, 45,000 black men are missing. In Philadelphia, there are 36,000 gone.[5] As a corollary, there are fewer and fewer older black men as well. In the wake of the police protests in Baltimore in 2015, a reporter asked a 28-year-old resident of the Sandtown neighborhood where the older men were. "'This is old here,' he said, pointing to himself. 'There ain't no more "Old Heads" anymore, where you been? They got big numbers or they in pine boxes.'"[6]

Age and class are significant factors here, and these have impacts on long-term health and life expectancy. Sixty percent of young black men who do not complete high school will be incarcerated by their middle thirties.[7] Among all black men ages 20 to 29, almost one in three is under some form of criminal justice oversight. According to the Bureau of Justice Statistics, one in three black men can expect to go to prison in his lifetime.[8] In cities like Chicago and Detroit that percentage is closer to 50 percent.

Mass Incarceration and Social Control

A graph of the rise in incarceration rates looks like an infectious-disease epidemic curve, with whopping acceleration beginning in the early 1970s after a hundred years of fairly flat rates.[9] Prior to the 1970s, the imprisonment rate in the United States was about 1 in 1,000, on par with the rest of the world. By 2000 the rate was 1 per 107, the highest in the world, with over 2.2 million people locked up and over 800,000 in pretrial detention. Roughly 3 percent of Americans (or about seven million people) are under the jurisdiction of the criminal justice system—locked up or on parole—on any given day.[10] And the rise of imprisonment rates has affected black and Latino communities disproportionately; the overall rate of white incarceration has not changed over the past forty years. Over 60 percent of incarcerated persons belong to racial and ethnic minorities. One in nine black men is incarcerated, compared to under two in one hundred of all white men.

Much of the rise in black incarceration can be attributed to three phenomena: aggressive policing practices, draconian drug laws, and harsh sentencing practices. It is also a direct result of the "law and order" and "tough on crime" movement that arose in the early 1970s when white politicians, like Nelson Rockefeller in New York and Richard Nixon nationally, began to call for tougher laws to preserve civil order—a code of sorts for keeping black people and other minorities stigmatized under the tight social control of the criminal justice system. During this period crime rates were rising, likely as a result of the baby boomers coming of age and the rapid urbanization of America after World War II. Although black incarceration rates had always been

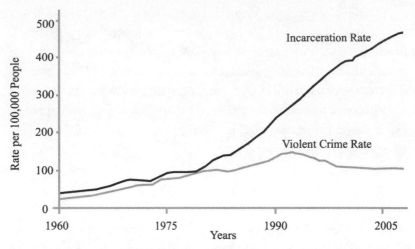

This graph illustrates the disconnect between violent crime rates and incarceration rates. While the incarceration rate has increased steadily over time, the violent crime rate has remained relatively stable, indicating that incarceration has had fairly low impact on violent crime. This is despite the United States' having the highest incarceration rate in the world. Source: CERP and Analysis of FBI and BJS Data.

higher than that of whites, under the new laws the black-white disparity in incarceration jumped.[11]

The rise in black imprisonment rates had no real correlation to the actual crime rates. In fact, while incarceration rates boomed after 1980, crime rates dropped. While some argue that the drop in the crime rate was a result of imprisonment, the best analyses suggest that if imprisonment had any effect at all, it was very small.[12] Studies show that while there is little to no relationship between the crime rate and the imprisonment rate, or between the crime rate and the proportion of black people in a state, there *is* a very strong relationship between the incarceration rate and the proportion of black people in a state. In other words, people go to prison in increasing numbers because they are black and poor, not because of a rise in the crime rate.[13] Aggressive policing, arrests, jailing, and imprisonment have replaced slavery and Jim Crow as the latest forms of social control in black (and Latino) communities—with stunning health consequences.[14]

Consequences of Mass Imprisonment

From a population health perspective there are pernicious consequences of imprisonment. They are best viewed from three perspectives: individual health, family health, and community health.

Prisons are unhealthy for individuals. Within prisons, HIV is about five times as prevalent as in the community.[15] Hepatitis C is nine to ten times more prevalent in prison than in the community and more deadly than HIV. Fifty-five percent of men and more than 70 percent of women in state prison have mental health problems.[16] Almost 70 percent of those incarcerated have diagnosable substance-use disorders, but fewer than 15 percent get any treatment.[17] Forty percent of incarcerated adults have one or more chronic condition, and as mandatory sentences have grown, the prison population has become older—and therefore more susceptible to a range of illnesses.[18] There is growing concern about the rates of traumatic brain injury among the prison population. Overcrowded facilities with poor sanitation and ventilation and inadequate services contribute to the ill health of the population. Suicide is responsible for one-third of prison deaths.[19]

For inmates, physical isolation and deprivation of human contact have become the norm. Control unit prisons, where prisoners are trapped in solitary confinement twenty-three hours daily, have sprung up across the country. The population of prisoners in solitary confinement exploded from a few hundred in the 1980s to almost 80,000 in 2010.[20] In August 2011 Juan Mendez, the United Nations special rapporteur on torture and other cruel, inhuman, or degrading treatment or punishment, concluded that even fifteen days in solitary confinement can cause long-standing psychological damage.[21] Those in isolation are seven times more likely to harm themselves.

But it is no safer for the 700,000 or so people per year who are released. Too many black parolees return to the communities of concentrated disadvantage that they came from, with little in the way of transitional support. Reentry turns out to be deadly across the board. The mortality rate of released prisoners is 3.5 times higher than that of the general population and 12.7 times higher during their first two weeks back in society.[22] Drug overdoses top the reasons for death, followed by heart disease, suicide, homicide, cancer, and motor vehicle accidents.

Imprisonment has a contagious effect on families and communities. When swaths of young men are pulled from their communities, families suffer. Because so many incarcerated men have drug addictions, mental illness, and infectious diseases, a huge burden is placed on their caregivers, usually women, when the men reenter society. Because there are few or no organized transitional social-support services for the ex-offender, the load falls onto the women's shoulders. It is no wonder that women caregivers of ex-convicts suffer from chronic health problems: 63 percent are smokers, 27 percent have hypertension, 34 percent report anxiety, and 36 percent report depression.[23] Community-based infectious disease outbreaks have been tied to prisons and jail returnees. Dangerous drug-resistant bacteria spread by former jail and prison inmates have spread in poor urban neighborhoods, posing a public health risk for the whole population. These bacteria resist treatment with commonly available antibiotics and have led to serious disease, hospitalizations, and deaths. In Chicago's West Side public housing units, the same neighborhoods devastated by blockbusting and by white and industry flight a half-century ago are now home to a deadly superbug: a pandemic strain of methicillin-resistant *Staphylococcus aureus* (MRSA).[24] This resistant bacteria was once found only in the sickest of hospitalized patients. Now it has jumped to the community, where it is spreading. A sevenfold increase in these infections was discovered in patients in area emergency rooms in 2007. Most were traced back to the Cook County Jail, an overcrowded, unsanitary environment where a reservoir of the bacteria has infected the inmates, who spread it when they are released.

The gender imbalances resulting from "missing" men are deleterious to community life and drive the chronic high poverty rates in these communities. The absence of men means that many children do not have an active father figure in their life. Women lack reliable partners to share the burden of childrearing and wage earning. The impact on these stresses on health and hope are devastating.

About 2.7 million children—including 1 in 14 African American children—have a parent behind bars, and that increases their own risk for future incarceration and ill health.[25] The effect on these children is devastating. Many children see no other paths for themselves than prison or death. In the book *There Are No Children Here*, author Alex Kotlowitz asked ten-year-old Lafayette Rivers what he wanted to be when he grew up.[26] Lafayette replied, "If I grow up, I'd like to be a bus driver." For those of us who have raised children in neighborhoods of concentrated advantage, this is a shocking response. But in America's abandoned neighborhoods, from a child's perspective, it is the honest truth.

Dostoevsky said, "The degree of civilization in a society can be judged by entering its prisons."[27] This is as true of its most disadvantaged communities. In America, these communities have been pummeled into permanent poverty and ill health by mass imprisonment. We can and must reverse this tide of decline.

8

IMMIGRATION STATUS AND HEALTH INEQUALITY

THE CASE OF TRANSPLANT

It is scandalous when one thinks about the people who live in a world in which they need not be hungry, in which they need not die without medical care, in which they need not be illiterate, they need not feel hopeless and miserable so much of the time, and yet they are.[1]

AMARTYA SEN

I have proposed that structural violence as a result of long-standing economic and public policies is responsible for low-status, low-life-expectancy neighborhoods across America. While neighborhood status and wealth are the major drivers of life expectancy, societal status, such as immigration status, contributes to premature mortality as well.

The United States has twenty-one million noncitizen residents, eleven million of whom are undocumented immigrants.[2] While some legal residents can eventually achieve health insurance eligibility, many remain uninsured. For those resident immigrants who are in the United States without legal permission, access to health insurance is near impossible. Federal and state policies have generally prohibited noncitizens from accessing public and private health insurance, with few exceptions. As a result, immigrants (legal and not) are three times as likely as citizens to be uninsured.[3] Even young adults who have been permitted to stay in the United States under the temporary amnesty program have been denied health insurance benefits available to citizens. It is unjust, in the wealthiest country in the world, that access to health care is denied simply because of one's immigration status.

Noncitizens contribute to the American safety net disproportion-ately to what they receive. Between 2000 and 2011, undocumented im-migrants contributed between $2.2 billion and $3.8 billion more than they withdrew from the Medicare Trust Fund each year.[4] That created a total surplus of $35.1 billion over the eleven-year span, staving off Medicare insolvency. But this is not simply an issue of money. It is a hu-man rights issue. When these noncitizens get a serious illness, they face early death, since they are denied health care. Sarai was one of these.

Sarai's Liver Transplant

Sarai was just 25 when her liver failed. Her life had been spiraling down-ward since she was diagnosed with Wilson's disease in the spring of 2013. Wilson's is a rare inherited disease that causes copper levels to rise in the blood. Over time the liver is infiltrated with copper. The damage is irreversible. Fluid builds up and swells the abdomen and feet. Poisons normally cleared by the liver accumulate in the body and cause mental confusion, bleeding disorders, and twitching of the hands and feet. Eventually the brain swells, and the patient dies.

The only cure is a liver transplant. When Sarai became sick with the first signs of liver failure, she was rushed to Stroger Hospital, the Chicago region's only public hospital. Her mother, Victoria, recounted her daughter's ordeal: "Well, they sent us to the hospital and since the beginning they told us that she needed a transplant but since she didn't have papers she didn't qualify for a transplant. First, Stroger said they didn't do them and then because of her migratory situation she didn't qualify for a transplant. The doctors from Rush [University Medical Center] came because Stroger works together with Rush and there are a lot of doctors from Rush there. And doctors from Rush told me that she didn't qualify for a transplant (because she was undocumented and uninsured.)[5]"

Despite the fact that Victoria worked full time at a job that provided health insurance, she had not purchased it. If you have no insurance and have liver failure, you cannot get an organ transplant anywhere in the United States. Despite the financial burden, Victoria was able to purchase health insurance that covered Sarai. Still, even after she had a new insurance card, Sarai was blocked from getting an appointment at another transplant center in Chicago, Northwestern Memorial Hospital.

Victoria explained, "But also at Northwestern, you see, they didn't want to give me the appointment. I called and... I already had the insurance.... They start to bombard you with questions that lead to if you're legal. And I told them no, no and 'how did you get the insurance?' they would ask and I said through my job. They said, 'Well, you don't have a valid social security number at your job so then your insurance is also not valid.'"[6]

After a call from Sarai's primary-care doctor, Northwestern relented and gave her an appointment for the fall of 2013. By then it was too late. Sarai died of liver failure in July.

Sarai's death is another example how inequity in health care access exacerbates the death gap, in this case for the millions of noncitizens who live and work in the United States but have no health insurance. While access to complex care such as a transplant is in some ways the tip of the iceberg, it shows how societal status drives inequality in health outcomes. There are people like Sarai all around us in the United States unable to access the most basic preventive health care. And yet for most Americans they remain invisible. Even when their suffering is apparent and visible to doctors and hospital staff, there is a refusal to break the rules. Or worse, a rush to judgment.

One of my patients, Roberto, is a 42-year-old man with kidney failure who moved his family to Illinois so he could pursue kidney care. In Texas there are no programs to provide ongoing kidney dialysis for the uninsured, so patients like Roberto either die or go to emergency rooms for care. When Roberto felt so sick that he could not go on, he drove to the nearest emergency room and waited until he received a lifesaving dialysis treatment. There among the swarms of patients and the bustle of doctors and nurses treating the ill, he lay on a gurney until he received the treatment that would allow him to function for a couple of days until the rising poisons made him ill again. That was a two-or-

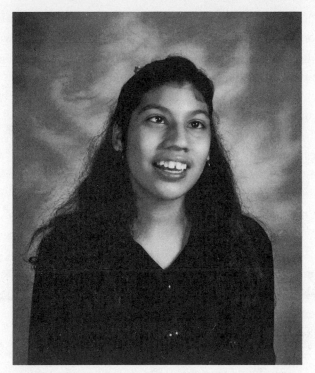

Sarai was 25 when she died waiting for an appointment for a transplant evaluation. Source: author's personal collection.

three-times-a-week experience for Roberto for two years. He ran back and forth to the hospital because routine lifesaving treatments, readily available to citizens, were denied him. His 18-year-old daughter Karina described how the nurses and doctors treated him as undeserving: "They were angry to see him back at the hospital even though it wasn't his fault that he was sick. The nurses told me to go back to Mexico, even though I am an American citizen."

If doctors and nurses are not willing to act on behalf of those who have been marginalized by our society because of social status, insurance status, race, or poverty, who will? Too often health care workers become self-appointed agents of structural violence, enforcers of unnatural and life-threatening rules about who gets access to health care in America. We fail to challenge our hospital or clinic policies that would deny care for the uninsured. Just as the police have become society's enforcers of structural racism in America's abandoned neighborhoods, administrators, nurses and doctors regularly assume the gatekeeper role to keep the uninsured and the poor from receiving all the care that is available in our institutions.

When the care is costly and complicated like kidney dialysis and transplantation for the uninsurable, the entrances of our institutions become even more impenetrable. We block (or in the case of Roberto and Karina, blame) patients who are seeking the care that we could provide. The issue of access to transplantation for the uninsured like Sarai and Roberto is even more poignant because federal law is clear that the transplant system is to be based on need, not money.

The National Organ Transplant Act

In 1984 Congress passed the National Organ Transplant Act, creating a rational, organized program of transplantation. Under the act, a federally appointed task force helped create a national organ allocation system "based on medical criteria that are publicly stated and fairly applied." The task force emphasized that organs should be distributed to those medically eligible "regardless of their ability to pay." The need for the act was driven by a desire for equity in the wake of controversial cases: in one, a businessman proposed to buy organs from individuals for resale purposes; in another, a rich Egyptian bought his way to the top of a transplant list. In order to encourage altruistic organ donation and equitable access, the act was clear that medical need, not financial circumstances, should dictate transplant allocation, under the assumption that people will donate organs only when they know that they will be allocated fairly.

Nevertheless, uninsured, undocumented patients like Sarai are routinely turned away early in the transplant evaluation process, which often consists of a barrage of medical and psychosocial testing undertaken to determine whether the patient will be a suitable caretaker of the organ. Regardless of their current medical condition, patients like Sarai rarely get to this step of the evaluation process, because of concerns about their inability to pay for the surgery and the long-term immunosuppressive therapy. Many potential undocumented and uninsured candidates are denied evaluation or allocation for financial reasons. Without transplants many patients die, some prematurely.

A Christmas Demonstration

In my role as the chief medical officer at Rush University Medical Center, I had not been familiar with the complex issues regarding access to transplantation in the undocumented until one late Friday afternoon, December 23, 2011. In addition to my administrative duties, I am a primary-care doctor and see patients every Friday. On this day I had seen patients all morning and into the afternoon. The staff had departed for the Christmas holiday, and I sat alone at the computer to complete my charting. As I slumped in front of the monitor, pecking at the keyboard, the telltale chime announced a new email.

"Hi doc, Wanted to give you a heads up," the subject line declared:

> Padre Jose Landaverde, the father of Our Lady of Guadalupe mission church is going to have a posada in front of Rush Hospital on Christmas Eve around 11am. They plan to march from their church that is located at 3442 W 26th Street starting at 10:15am. This is pretty dramatic because it's a far walk and cold, they have a number of extremely sick members in their church, and the future seems rather bleak, especially where undocumented, uninsured families are concerned.... We will be joining him to request a meeting with the Hospital leadership to address concerns of the community.

The email went on a bit more about Rush and its insensitivity to health issues among the undocumented. The note ended, "I guess that's what Rush gets for blowing off the community. Besos y abrazos, Emma."

Emma was a well-known community activist. She had been one of the leaders of a 150,000-person march for immigration reform to Chicago's Loop in 2007, a protest that put Chicago at the center for the drive for justice for undocumented residents. That same year, she and her husband, the Reverend Walter "Slim" Coleman, had provided refuge to an undocumented immigrant and hunger striker, Elvira Arellano, in their church for eight months, a case that brought national attention to the plight of the undocumented.

Today, however, they were planning a demonstration at my hospital. And not just any kind of demonstration, a posada, a Mexican Christmas tradition in which parishioners reenact Joseph and Mary's search for shelter for the birth of Jesus. From December 16 to December 24, parishioners go door to door singing carols. Generally on Christmas Eve the final destination is the parish church, but this group was planning to come to my hospital instead.

Attached to the email from Emma was a leaflet describing the march and giving the phone number of a Father Landaverde, the organizer. I decided to call him.

"Hey, Father," I said after identifying myself, "I understand that you are holding a demonstration at Rush tomorrow. Can I ask you why?"

"Yes, Doctor," he said in Spanish-inflected English. "Rush refused to treat a patient."

"What's the patient's name?" I asked.

"Elfego Alvarez. Mr. Alvarez has amyloidosis, and he needs a liver transplant to live. His mother died of the disease, and his two brothers have it as well. Rush turned Mr. Alvarez down."

Familial amyloidosis is an autosomal dominant disease, which means that either parent can pass it on to his or her children. An abnormal protein made by the liver invades the heart, nerves, intestines, and kidneys. It eventually strangles the organs, causing a painful death. Most patients with amyloidosis are dead by the age of forty. No medications exist to treat it. As in Sarai's case, the only possible cure for a patient with amyloidosis is a liver transplant. Without a liver transplant the disease is 100 percent fatal.

While Rush and other transplant centers are required to provide charity care, transplantation services are often excluded from it. The reason is that, unlike many other treatments, transplantation requires a lifetime of very expensive antirejection medications, which over time can cost hundreds of thousands of dollars. Most poor, uninsured, and undocumented patients are excluded because their families cannot raise the money. At Rush and many other transplant hospitals, patients might have to raise $150,000 before they are allowed to be evaluated for a transplant. Sarai's mom recalled how impossible this is for any family: "Some tell you $250,000 and others tell you it can cost you up to $500,000. When can you fundraise even half of $100,000? Simply... well, you can't even fundraise for $10,000."

But even as most of the poor and uninsured are denied transplants, in the United States about 20 percent of the organs for transplant come from the uninsured. In Chicago, 30 percent of donated organs come from the uninsured, and 3 percent come from noncitizens.[7] Transplantation is a profitable business, and the transplant centers and the pharmaceutical companies make excellent margins for providing the services. This arrangement is blatantly exploitative.

To compound the problem, there is a large racial gap in transplants as well, with whites more likely to get transplant evaluation and allocation than blacks and Latinos, independent of insurance. Justice and federal law dictate that access to transplants should be more equitable. The transplant literature shows that when the poor receive transplants and have insurance coverage for long-term care, they do as well at organ stewardship as those with more financial means.

A Demonstration for Transplants

I decided to meet the demonstrators and hear what they had to say. It was a blustery, gray December day. The icy wind down Harrison Street stung my face. A gaggle of about thirty demonstrators lined the sidewalks. The Rush security guards were keeping them from approaching the building. One teenage boy with a mop of black hair and a peach-fuzz mustache was playing a snare drum. A doe-eyed, serious-looking teenage girl with straight black hair strummed a guitar. Standing with a battery-powered megaphone was Emma. Emma was in her late fifties, short and trim with straight black hair and a gray fedora. Her dark eyes gleamed when she saw me.

"Hey, doc. Your security guys won't let us near the front door."

Next to Emma, leaning on his cane with a lit Marlboro dangling from his lips, stood her husband. Slim was six-foot-four, his back bent with arthritis, a deeply creased chain smoker's face, light blue eyes, tobacco-stained teeth, and a silver-streaked red goatee. He wore a loosely fitting food-stained black shirt with a white clerical collar, open at the neck. Draped over his lanky frame was a wash-weary navy blue hoodie with a faded image of Our Lady of Guadalupe on the back.

Before Slim had become a Methodist minister, he had been a street-hardened community organizer in the Uptown neighborhood, fighting the infamous Democratic political machine. Born in West Texas and educated at Harvard, Slim had come to Chicago in the 1960s as a civil rights, Black Panther, union, and antiwar organizer. Ultimately he settled into organizing the white working-class people who had migrated to Uptown from West Virginia and Tennessee. He had been known as a clenched-fist organizer who encouraged his minions in the Uptown People's Coalition to seek out the Democratic machine thugs on their street corners and "beat the shit outta them."[8] His organizing skills helped elect a Democratic antimachine reformer as Uptown's alderman. Now he spent his efforts working on issues of social justice from Lincoln Methodist Church in a Mexican neighborhood not far from Rush. Many of its parishioners were undocumented and had no access to health care.

I walked up to Lauris, the chief of security, and pulled him aside. Lauris was a giant of a man. He towered over the demonstrators, many of whom were Mexican and children. "Let's invite them into the lobby," I said.

"But they have a bullhorn and musical instruments!"

"We'll ask them not to play them," I replied.

Satisfied, he allowed me to invite the crowd in. I put my arm around Slim's waist, and he leaned on me as I escorted him in. The warm lobby was a welcome contrast to the outdoor cold.

Just then another group of demonstrators arrived. This crowd numbered about forty people, men and women, boys and girls, old and young. Many were carrying signs, posters, and banners with pictures of sick people. One large banner proclaimed "HERMANOS ALVAREZ" in bold letters and pictured the three Alvarez brothers, standing together, almost life sized. Another pictured a woman in a hospital bed with words emblazoned in red marker, pleading for a bone marrow transplant. All of the patients were in need of transplants. And from the looks on the faces of the crowd, many sick people had made the march. I could detect the copper-colored faces of patients with renal failure. As the kidneys fail, poisons accumulate in the body and stain the skin. One man in particular caught my eye. He was thin and sickly, a gray-faced, sad-eyed, bone-thin man. In his arms he cradled a plastic baby Jesus dressed in a white lace baptismal gown. I recognized him from his picture on the banner. He was Elfego Alvarez, who needed a liver transplant. Next to him was a short brown-skinned minister with white clerical collar under a blue parka and red scarf. His hair, jet black and pomaded, was combed straight back. He was speaking in Spanish to a Univision television crew who had arrived on the scene.

"We are here to ask for *posada* from Rush Hospital and other medical centers. Do not value material things over people's lives. If you do it's a sin. We are here to ask for *posada* for the following people," and he listed a group of names, presumably of those in the crowd. "They are being condemned, simply for being undocumented.... We are here to ask Rush Hospital to take care of all these families."

This was Father José Landaverde. I later learned that he was a Salvadoran refugee who had come to Chicago as an immigrant teen, was nurtured by Catholic nuns, and found his way into the ministry, where he was active in social justice issues. He presided over a storefront Episcopal church on 26th Street in the heart of the Mexican La Villita neighborhood.

When he was done speaking with the press, I invited him into the lobby, too, and listened to the patients he brought with him. I heard story after story from patients in need of transplant. The most compelling was that of Elefego Arroyo and his brother Lorenzo, both with amyloidosis. A third brother, Francisco, had recently completed a transplant at Rush. He was a US citizen and had Blue Cross Blue Shield insurance. Elefego was a patient at Stroger Hospital, down the street from Rush. His brother was a patient at the University of Illinois Hospital, also in the neighborhood.

There was another patient, George Martinez, a studious-looking young man with black hair and horn-rimmed glasses, who needed a kidney transplant. He had been brought to the US at the age of one and developed renal failure at sixteen. He was covered at that time by public insurance, but he was never offered a transplant anywhere. He was now twenty-three, as American as apple pie but undocumented and uninsured. George described his dilemma: "They told me that I should go back to Mexico to get a transplant. But Mexico is a foreign country to me. I have been in Chicago all my life."

I told Father Landaverde that Rush would evaluate Elefego for a liver transplant (he eventually received one). I also agreed to invite him back to open a dialogue with the senior leadership at Rush. But, I said, the other transplant centers will have to do their fair share as well. I promised to reach out to them. I spoke to the leaders at the University of Illinois and asked them to evaluate Lorenzo for a liver transplant. I asked Loyola University Medical Center to evaluate George for a kidney transplant. These would be humanitarian gestures, as both men were uninsured. Both centers refused.

Hunger Strikes for Transplants

The summer of 2012 brought new activity from Father Landaverde's church. The number of patients needing transplants grew from five to fifty as undocumented patients with end-stage organ disease heard about his ministry. One of the congregants proposed that the members of the congregation go on a hunger strike. It lasted twenty-one days, and the strikers were arrested for blocking the lobbies at the University of Illinois and Loyola Hospitals. The strike ended when both centers said that they would take one patient for evaluation.

Six months later, George Martinez received his kidney transplant, from his mother, who surely would have donated it when he was sixteen. Still, at twenty-three he was finally free from the three days a week of dialysis. The University of Illinois Hospital evaluated Lorenzo, but by then his amyloidosis was too advanced.

The summer of 2013 brought another hunger strike and demonstrations and arrests in front of Northwestern Memorial Hospital, the largest transplant center in Chicago, spurred in part by Sarai's plight and death. After Sarai's funeral, the hunger strikers carried a casket with her name on it seven miles from the church to Northwestern. They held a mock funeral in front of the doors. The incident received national and international media attention. The next week I called Father

Landaverde and asked him to call off his hunger strike. I promised to call a meeting of all the transplant centers and the community.

A Breakthrough

I invited the transplant centers, civic groups, some politicians, and the community representatives to convene at Rush. The transplant centers were wary, afraid of negative publicity. After many phone calls, I promised no publicity, just conversation. I decided to divide the meeting in two parts. This first part would be a dialogue with Father Landaverde, Rev. Coleman, and other community members. The second half would be a discussion with the transplant centers, Mexican consulate representatives, and politicians about how to respond to the need. I was worried because the transplant centers were so anxious about Father Landaverde and his aggressive activism.

I was not apprehensive about him at all. He and I had developed a cordial and respectful relationship. I never promised anything beyond listening to him and his congregation and trying to work with the other centers to find solutions to what seemed to be an intractable problem. I had visited him and his congregation in their storefront church. After that first posada demonstration, he never again held a demonstration at Rush, I believe in part because we listened and tried to help.

The meeting was held on August 27, 2013, in a large conference room at Rush with a row of windows along one wall. Across the way we could see the old Cook County Hospital, where many of the transplant petitioners had received care. Representatives from the Mexican consulate, Stroger Hospital, the organ procurement organization, state and local politicians, community groups, and all but one of the local transplant centers were present around a long U-shaped table.

A hum of conversation was filling the air when Father Landaverde walked in. He carried a brown burlap book bag with Che Guevara's image stenciled in black on the side. With him was a group of young people from his church, all of whom needed transplantation. He made the case for fairness and justice for the undocumented and uninsured. Then some of his congregants spoke. George Martinez thanked Loyola for allowing him to receive a kidney but decried how long it took to get the attention he deserved. Bianca, a 21-year-old with kidney failure, noted that it had taken demonstrations and hunger strikes to get the attention of transplant centers. After the public meeting, administrators of the transplant centers met with the politicians to discuss ways to solve the dilemma.

We discussed the possibility of getting the state to pay for kidney transplants. Illinois is one of eleven states that provide lifetime dialysis services for the undocumented. A kidney transplant would free an individual from being tethered to a machine for life. I asked, "Wouldn't it be more effective to allow these patients to get transplants than to condemn them to a lifetime of dialysis?" It would be cheaper in the long run, because one or two years of dialysis treatments is more costly than a kidney transplant.

The meeting ended without a solution but with a sense of hope. Those in the room were touched by the stories from the patients, all of whom were in their twenties. We agreed to keep talking. These talks led to new legislation and new opportunities for these patients.

A Door Opens

One year after Sarai's death, after the hunger strikes, after meetings and discussions, a law sponsored by the Latino caucus passed the Illinois State Assembly and the Senate and was signed by the governor. This legislation allows the undocumented to receive kidney transplants and lifetime medications, paid with state funds. Unfortunately, the current governor, a Tea Party Republican, has refused to fund the program. But patchwork private programs have been popped up as well. One funded by the American Kidney Fund provides insurance-premium support to the undocumented with end-stage kidney disease. The passage of the Affordable Care Act allows the undocumented with preexisting conditions to purchase health insurance directly from insurance companies. With these two initiatives, many previously uninsured noncitizen patients in Illinois have been evaluated and received access to transplants. A new fund, the Illinois Transplant Fund, was created to pay the insurance premiums for uninsured transplant patients.

One patient, Martin, age 28, who received a kidney from his brother at my hospital, wrote me afterward, "After seven years finally I am going to be able to have a happy Christmas with my family, thanks to all of you for giving me this special gift of a second chance at living. I want to share to all of you that now I see life just as if I was born again. Thanks to the kidney transplant, my esteem is back up and I also decided to study and now have obtained my GED."

While this is a hopeful note, inequality cannot be fixed one disease at a time, one hospital at a time, one insurance policy at a time, in one city at a time. Noncitizens need full and unfettered access to health care. Yes, we are required as doctors and nurses to do what we can on behalf of our patients, no matter their circumstances. But we also have to be willing to take on the structural violence: the laws and policies that prematurely kill patients like Sarai by denying access to care to a whole class of indivudals. Maybe Sarai would never have qualified for a transplant. Maybe an organ would not have come available in time to save her life. Maybe Sarai would not have survived the surgery and the postoperative period. But Sarai was not even allowed the chance to be evaluated for transplant because of her citizenship. The death gap is not an abstract concept. There are people like Sarai in every town and city in America. For me, it is palpable, poignant, and personal—because I bear some responsibility for Sarai's premature death at the age of 25. My hospital's doctors refused to evaluate her initially because she had no insurance. If we believe that equal access to health care is a fundamental human right, Sarai's story should motivate us to make equitable universal health care a reality. We're not there yet.

PART 3
HEALTH CARE
INEQUALITY

THE US HEALTH CARE SYSTEM: SEPARATE AND UNEQUAL

Our society ensures that large numbers of people, in the United States and out of it, will be simultaneously put at risk for disease and denied access to care. In fact, the spectacular successes of biomedicine have in many instances further entrenched medical inequalities.[1]

PAUL FARMER

The US healthcare system provides unequal care. Just as life expectancy is determined by which neighborhood you live in, for many Americans what hospital or doctor you can see is influenced by neighborhood, insurance, race, and ethnicity. And if you live in a high-mortality neighborhood, a trip to the local hospital might just be a matter of life and death.

There are three major reasons why health care delivery in the United States is not equitable. The first is that health care is treated as commodity, not a right. The poor (with or without insurance) living in neighborhoods of concentrated disadvantage often have more limited access to quality health care.[2] Those who are uninsured and underinsured experience great difficulty accessing needed care.[3] Minorities and the poor are less likely to have private health insurance than white middle-class Americans.[4] When minorities and the poor do have insurance, it is more likely to be one of the publicly funded insurance policies that not all hospitals and doctors accept. The second reason is that minorities sometimes get different treatment for the same illness from what whites get, regardless of insurance. Health care providers' implicit racial bias and patients' mistrust may be the causes of this differential treatment.[5] The third reason why health care delivery is unequal is that the health care institutions that serve the poor in general suffer from cash and capital shortages. Neighborhoods of concentrated advantage where people with better insurance live have better-resourced hospitals and clinics than poor neighborhoods do.

This is how structural violence works within the fabric of the health care system. It is not as if great care cannot be delivered in underserved settings. It is, every day. But it is inconsistent or constrained by a lack of resources. Thus minorities and poor people die disproportionally as a result of an unfairly structured American health care system.

The Deadly Divide

Take breast cancer care. It is a gruesome fact that in the United States, black women are 40 percent more likely to die from breast cancer than white women. While black and white American women now develop breast cancer at the same rates (something that was not always the case), more black women will die of the disease.[6]

Why does this particular death gap exist? An oncologist will tell you that black women first seek treatment with larger, more deadly, later-stage breast cancers.[7] But the truth is that the breast cancer death gap is not just a biological phenomenon but a consequence of structural violence. A woman's neighborhood can determine whether she will survive breast cancer or die from it.

It would be grisly enough if breast cancer were the only disease that discriminated. It is not. From heart disease to hepatitis C, depression to diabetes, blacks throughout the United States suffer higher rates of illness and death than whites. It is tough to name many diseases that do not discriminate by race, place, and poverty. But breast cancer is a disease that demonstrates vividly how structural violence is woven into neighborhood fabric, especially in black communities.

The Missed Breast Cancer

The key to unlocking the inequity in breast cancer mortality came from a radiology reading room on the top floor of Mercy Hospital on Martin Luther King Jr. Drive on Chicago's South Side. The room was dark except for the projected image of a mammogram. Amid the cool gray background of fatty breast tissue was an unmistakable irregular-shaped mass, its speculated white tentacles invading the surrounding tissue— a telltale sign of advanced breast cancer. It was as obvious as a ticking bomb.

Dr. Paula Grabler, a radiologist specializing in reading mammograms and diagnosing breast cancer, was then the director of breast imaging services. At most of the other small hospitals that served South Side African American communities, mammograms were read not by specialists but by general radiologists. Too often cancers were evident but missed. This case was no different.

"She was a middle-aged African American woman," Dr. Grabler recalled.[8] "The patient had been seen in the past at a small South Side hospital and had a screening mammogram that was reported to be normal. Months later she came to me with a lump in her breast. I asked to get a copy of the prior mammogram and there it was: a large, very obvious breast cancer."

Grabler typically removes mammograms from the view box when she meets with patients. She does not want the image of the cancer to shock the patient. "But on this particular day, I forgot to," she said.

The patient gasped when she saw the large white mass that exploded from the gray background of the x-ray. "How did they miss it?" she asked. It was a glaring mistake that could cost her her life.

"I honestly don't know," Grabler replied. But she did know. The doctor who read her mammogram was not an expert. He was an itinerant radiologist who read all types of x-rays. Detecting breast cancer early requires meticulous attention to detail. Trained experts who read mammograms find six times more breast cancers than general radiologists do.[9] In Chicago, most of the breast centers that are near or in the black wards do not have such specialists. Cancers are missed. Women die.

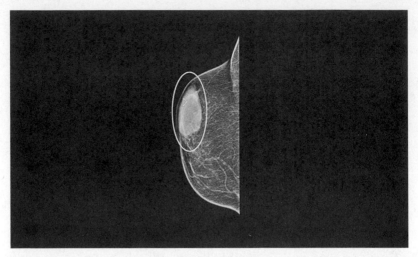

An obvious breast cancer on a mammogram. The patient presented with a lump in her breast; the prior mammogram had been read as normal. Sometimes the cause of racial disparities in health care can be as banal as an inexperienced or busy doctor missing cancer. Source: author's personal collection.

That missed breast cancer held the key to understanding an aspect of premature mortality: access to screening is important for finding breast cancer early—but the quality of that screening is even more critical. We found a screening facility serving Chicago's black community that found two breast cancers for every thousand women screened, when the correct number should have been at least six.[10] More than half were missed. Add to this injury the insult a black woman feels later when she goes to see a doctor with a bad cancer and is told that her genetics are at fault.

Institutional racism as a structural cause of increased mortality can sometimes be as banal as a poorly qualified doctor missing a cancer in a poorly run mammography center. In a Chicago study of missed breast cancers, poor women, minority women, and publicly insured women were significantly more likely than well-insured white women to have their cancers missed (they were there on the mammogram on a lookback.)[11] Socially disadvantaged women (poor, minority, and un-insured) are significantly more likely to have a cancer missed on mammography because they are more likely to receive care at substandard facilities, in segregated neighborhoods, than advantaged women are.[12]

Even if women of color do everything right—get screened, schedule follow-up appointments—they can still fare worse than white women simply by virtue of where they live. This is not just a product of poverty, though poverty itself is a big predictor of inequity. There are plenty of poor white women in Chicago, but there is not one poor white Chicago neighborhood.[13] Poor white women can get their breast care in the same neighborhood hospitals as the more wealthy women in their neighborhoods. This is structural violence and institutionalized racism at work. Women living in Chicago's neighborhoods of concentrated advantage are 37 times more likely have ready access to a "breast center of excellence" than women living in high-poverty neighborhoods.[14] This maldistribution of resources did not occur by chance.

The Spread of Racial Disparity

None of this mattered when there were no effective treatments for breast cancer. From the mid-1930s, when breast cancer mortality was first measured in the United States, until the early 1980s, when screening mammography and new chemotherapy agents were shown to be effective at reducing mortality, there were no black-to-white or rich-to-poor gaps in breast cancer mortality.[15] But in the early 1990s, as breast cancer became more amenable to new treatments, the breast cancer death rate for white women across the United States began to plummet.[16] The death rate for black women in Chicago did not budge.[17]

The improvement for white women was easy to comprehend. Years of effort to raise awareness about the importance of regular mammography screenings coupled with improvements in technology and the emergence of specialists like Grabler meant that more cancers were detected early. Meanwhile, advances in treatment further increased survival rates.

But it was here that a new racial death divide emerged. It grew from a sliver to a chasm over the next twenty years. Poor women, and specifically poor black women, were not getting the same quality of breast cancer care as wealthier and white women. Researchers have described this growing racial gap in cancer mortality as the "amenability factor."[18] As cancers such as breast cancer become more amenable to treatment interventions, racial cancer survival disparities widen because poor minority women do not have easy access to the lifesaving cures.[19]

Inequality in Quality

In 2007, 160-plus doctors, researchers, and community activists in Chicago convened the Metropolitan Chicago Breast Cancer Task Force to investigate the gap and decide how to close it. We analyzed the data. We drilled into the deaths. We held focus groups of black and Latina women on the South and West Sides. We heard their stories of fragmented and disrespectful health care in their communities. We released a report.[20] It confirmed that access to quality of care was responsible for the wide racial gaps in breast cancer mortality. The report also made thirty-seven recommendations for closing the gap.

Yet breast cancer researchers scoffed. They clung to the usual genetic and biological explanations. We fought back, pointing out the structural components of the death gap, both in Chicago and nationwide. Chicago's gap was twice as large as the national gap and seven times larger than the gap in New York City, suggesting that geography is a significant variable.[21] Cities like Memphis and every major Texas city had even larger breast cancer death gaps than Chicago's.[22] In Detroit, black and white women had the same terrible mortality rates. The cities with the greatest breast cancer death gaps were also the ones with the largest dissimilarity index scores, denoting advanced degrees of racial segregation.[23] Moreover, biology cannot explain the variability in the racial death rates in cities within the same state. For example, in Los Angeles black women are 71 percent more likely to die from breast cancer than whites. In Sacramento and San Francisco this gap does not exist.[24]

A Map and a Story

The task force published a map of Chicago showing the communities with the highest breast cancer mortality. Twenty-three were black communities and one was white. All were located on the West and South Sides. All the black communities were neighborhoods of concentrated

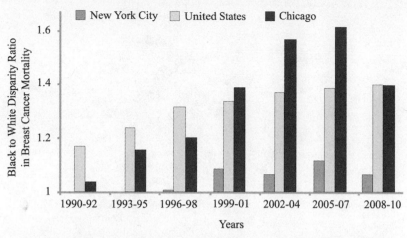

Disparity ratios in breast cancer mortality between white and black women across New York City, the United States, and Chicago from 1990 to 2010 show that geography, more than biological and genetic factors, influences women's mortality. Source: Metropolitan Chicago Breast Cancer Task Force.

poverty and disadvantage.[25] In mostly black neighborhoods, not one hospital has earned the American College of Radiology's seal of approval for breast imaging centers. Only one hospital in a high-mortality black neighborhood has been certified by the American College of Surgeons' Commission on Cancer as a cancer treatment center. In contrast, in the white wards there are fourteen cancer accredited hospitals. This was a bleak picture of the structural nature of racial inequality.

It's one thing to look at disparity on a map. It's another to hear from the women who try to navigate the fractured system of care. Chicago and other cities have a hodgepodge of public and private hospitals and clinics, with little communication between them and poor coordination of care. Barbara Akpan is a retired nurse in Chicago. After her breast cancer diagnosis and treatment at an academic medical center, she began serving as a volunteer community advocate for other African American women on the South Side. Her observations reinforce the notion that inequality in the quality of breast cancer care was failing women.

"Many of the women I work with are afraid," she said. "They do not trust the health care system. Many of the clinics and hospitals they go to do not provide the best care, or they simply give them the wrong

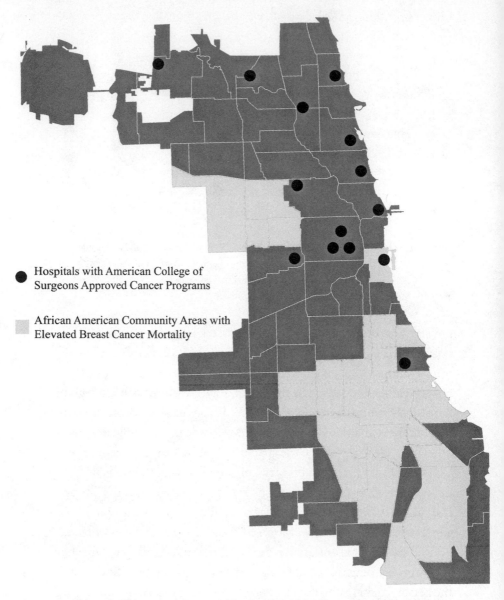

Hospitals with American College of
Surgeons Approved Cancer Programs

African American Community Areas with
Elevated Breast Cancer Mortality

In Chicago's African American neighborhoods with high mortality for female breast
cancer, there are few hospitals with American College of Surgeons–approved cancer
programs. Consequently, black women with breast cancer concerns have to either
travel for care or receive care at nonapproved cancer treatment sites. This map depicts
how health inequality is structured into the geography of a region. Source: http://
link.springer.com/article/10.1007/s10552-009-9419-7.

information. It's hard to overcome the mistrust. For women in the southland—Ford Heights, Chicago Heights, Harvey, poor areas on the South Side—access to mammography screening sites is really poor," says Akpan. "Women are falling through the gap—they don't know where to go."[26]

When we traveled around Chicago and other cities, showed audiences of black women the mortality curves illustrating the black breast cancer death gap, and gave our explanations, they cried. We had validated something they knew to be true: the systems that served them were often inadequate. They cried because our data told them that the breast cancer death gap was a system problem and not a problem within black women. Their reactions galvanized us to focus on fixing the system.

Because the mortality gap was structural, we needed hospitals to work together to improve care for black women. We identified hospitals with undertrained mammography technicians and radiologists and arranged free continuing-education courses. We met with CEOs to share their hospital's quality data and make recommendations for improvement. But this was not going to improve care fast enough. If a small inner-city hospital lacked the expertise to provide comprehensive breast cancer care, no amount of quality improvement would remedy it. But what if we could move women from poor institutions to good ones?

Navigating to Quality

We hired health "navigators." These were community health workers and nurses who could direct women to high-quality hospitals for screening and treatment. We solicited breast cancer services from all the region's top hospitals. Most obliged. The navigators guide their clients into care at the city's highest-quality medical centers even when they are two hours and two bus transfers away. Sometimes the navigators battle with the local doctors to wrest the patient into better care.

Gerri Murrah is typical of the patients navigated. She was 60 and developed a sore lump in her breast in 2015. Not having a primary-care physician, she had gone to her local emergency room. The doctor didn't even consider cancer; Gerri was given antibiotics and sent home. Luckily, Murrah knew something was wrong and went to a different clinic and requested a mammogram. The results were suspicious. Murrah was assigned to a surgeon at a neighborhood hospital. This surgeon, not a breast specialist, made two bungles: Instead of doing a needle biopsy, he surgically removed the lump—a painful and unnecessary procedure. Then, without informing Murrah of the stage of her breast cancer (stage III), he recommended an unneeded mastectomy. When DeShauna Dickens, one of the task force navigators, finally connected with Murrah, she referred Murrah to the University of Chicago Hospital for a second opinion. There, Murrah learned she had other options that would preserve her breast.

"DeShauna came in just in time to stop me from having my breast cut off," she says, in an *O, the Oprah Magazine* interview.[27]

There are setbacks. Not all women respond. Not all institutions have the will to better their conditions. Some facilities were deplorable, such as the mammography facility in the Washington Park neighborhood's Provident Hospital, which the task force staff visited in 2014. The room that was used to develop mammography films had a sewer manhole cover in the middle of the floor and was suffused with noxious sewer fumes. The path to improve quality and reduce mortality can be slow and painful.

The Breast Cancer Quality Consortium

Yet progress has been made. The grassroots team persuaded 160 health care providers across the state, including every Chicago hospital, to share their data, such as tumor detection rates and follow-up rates. Slow improvements in quality were made even in the poorly performing hospitals. In 2013, after seven years of work, the black-white breast cancer death gap in Chicago had narrowed by 35 percent.[28] While the exact reasons for the improvement in the mortality gap are not easy to tease out, in no other metropolitan area of the United States has that death gap been reduced. The reduction in black breast-cancer deaths in Chicago shows that mortality inequities caused by structural violence are fixable. Focused and deliberate work directed at equalizing the health care system can save lives. Racial disparity can be reduced—and possibly eliminated. "We don't need a magic bullet to fix this," says Dr. Patricia Ganz, a member of the Breast Cancer Research Foundation Scientific Advisory Board and professor of medicine and public health at UCLA. "We just need to give black women the same standard of care."[29]

Implicit Bias Contributes to Unequal Care

While the story of the Chicago breast cancer death gap has had early success, in too many areas and on too many levels we are still dealing with the most basic inequities and prejudices. Bias, even if unconscious, affects individual physicians and their treatment decisions. This is unsettling but true. While most doctors do not exhibit explicit racial bias, such as refusing to treat certain patients because of their race, on tests of implicit bias they, too, show unconscious preferences for whites over dark-skinned faces. The Implicit Association Test is a widely used test of social cognition. More than 70 percent of the millions of Americans who have taken it exhibit a subconscious preference for whites over blacks.[30] Physicians score similarly.

An ingenious 1999 experiment showed how unconscious bias affects clinical decision making. Thousands of doctors were asked to test their clinical acumen by reviewing the medical history given by a performer who acted out the symptoms of a potential cardiac syndrome on film.[31] There were eight elderly patients. Four were men: two white and two black. Four were women: two white and two black. Physicians were asked to recommend a cardiac workup based on the clinical information the patients relayed. In addition, physicians were told whether the patient was insured or uninsured.

The results were not surprising. Based on the gender, race, and insurance status of the patient, doctors recommended entirely different medical workups. Men of both races were more likely to be referred for angiograms to evaluate symptoms of chest pain. But blacks of both genders were less likely than the whites to be referred for the full cardiac workup. Those who were noted to be insured were more likely to be referred for a full workup as well. While this was an experiment and not real clinical care, unconscious bias in health care delivery seems to be a real phenomenon.

In an eye-opening 2002 report on health care disparities, the Institute of Medicine found "strong but circumstantial evidence for the role of bias, stereotyping, and prejudice" in perpetuating racial health disparities.[32] Some research suggests that there is a direct relationship among physicians' implicit bias, mistrust on the part of black patients, and clinical outcomes.[33] In a prospective study of older adults, patients who experienced discrimination in health care more than once yearly were twice as likely to have a disability four years later than cohort members who suffered no discrimination.[34]

What needs to be done to address implicit bias in medicine? Awareness is a start. Mandatory bias testing and cultural intelligence training have been proposed. But it requires day-to-day interactions between people of different backgrounds to break the implicit boundaries that prevent deeper understanding.[35] And that's necessary, but fair. But bias is only a piece of the story.

Having No Insurance Is Bad for Your Health

Another major factor driving inequitable care is lack of health insurance. Uninsured adults are far more likely than those with insurance to postpone or forgo health care altogether. Twenty-five percent of adults without coverage say that they went without care in the past year because of its cost, compared to 4 percent of adults with private insurance coverage. Moreover, 55 percent of uninsured adults do not have a regular place to go when they are sick or need medical advice.[36] When uninsured patients get injured or develop a chronic disease that requires follow up, they are less likely than those with coverage to actually obtain all the services that are recommended.[37] Blacks and Latinos are more likely to be uninsured than whites, which only increases the burdens of health care inequity borne in neighborhoods of concentrated poverty. Prior to the Affordable Care Act, an estimated 45,000 residents died each year due to a lack of insurance, or one person every twelve minutes. If being uninsured was a cause of death, it would be the tenth most common one in the United States.[38] The next chapter will deal further with the issue of health insurance.

Apartheid Hospitals

Once people do get insurance, there is no guarantee they will get good treatment. As Nobel Prize winner Angus Deaton has noted, "Hospitals in the United States are run on something close to an apartheid basis with few white patients in the hospitals that treat mostly African Americans and vice versa."[39] Hospitals in which the majority of patients served are minorities have higher mortality rates across the board, whether from trauma, cardiac surgery, or general surgery procedures. In fact, as the percentage of minority patients served increases at an institution, so do the mortality rates across many conditions. There seems to be a direct correlation between the proportion of minority patients served by a hospital and death rates.[40]

Take trauma care as an example. Trauma centers that serve mostly minority patients have higher mortality rates than those that serve mostly white patients. There is a gradation of trauma mortality based on the percentage of minority patients served by the trauma center. Those trauma hospitals with fewer than 25 percent minority patients have 60 percent better trauma survival rates than trauma hospitals with more than 50 percent minority patients. Hospitals with 25–50 percent minority patients have trauma mortalities in between the two.[41] Why would this be? Trauma centers require specific levels of physician and other staff coverage, and they require periodic rigorous certification. Shouldn't this attention and regulation lead to better care, regardless of race and ethnicity? There are only two possibilities. One is that trauma severity or high-risk conditions are more prevalent among patients in institutions that serve mostly minorities. However, even when severity of illness is controlled for, minority trauma centers have 37 percent higher mortality rates than those serving mostly whites. The other possibility is that the care is actually unequal. I have shown how this is true for breast cancer care. It seems to be true for many conditions.

What hospital you attend is literally a matter of life and death. In general, hospitals and clinics where many minority patients receive

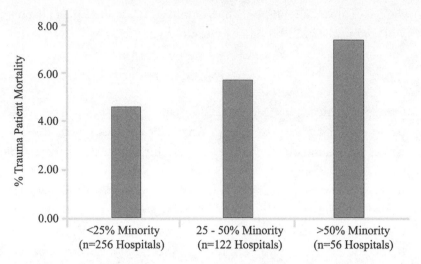

Hospitals that serve more minorities tend to have higher patient mortality rates than hospitals serving fewer minorities, reflecting the lack of resources and disparity in health care for the different racial populations. This figure shows how the likelihood of dying from trauma increases in hospitals that serve more minority patients. This is an example of structural racism. Source: *Archives of Surgery* 147 (2012).

care are lower quality than those that serve white populations, whether for medical or surgical conditions.[42] Further, hospitals treating a higher proportion of black patients have higher mortality rates for many surgical procedures. In addition, these hospitals have higher mortality rates independent of race: both black patients and white patients have higher mortality in hospitals with mostly black patients than their racial counterparts in other centers.[43] The federal Center for Medicare and Medicaid Services recently created a national star ranking system for hospitals, to allow consumers a means to assess hospital quality. A hospital can be ranked from five stars to one star, with five stars denoting a very high quality hospital with lower mortality and one star being a low-quality hospital with high mortality.[44] In practice, star rankings vary by the whiteness of the hospital's clentele. Five- and four-star hospitals in America serve patient populations that are predominantly white. One- and two-star hospitals in America serve predominantly minority paitients and very few whites.

This is true for care at clinics as well as hospitals. The doctors who work at clinics that care for predominantly black and other minority populations are less likely to be board certified, have less access to specialty consultation, and work in more chaotic conditions. It is not a matter of the patients' race or ethnicity. Hospitals and clinics in poor neighborhoods, those that serve uninsured populations or those on Medicaid, often do not have enough resources to provide the very best care.[45] What seems at first blush to be a racial disparity is actually a consequence of structural violence and institutionalized racism. Just follow the money.

Let's compare the cash situations at two Chicago hospitals, both trauma centers. During my decade at Mount Sinai Hospital, located in a low-income black neighborhood, 20 percent of the patients had no insurance. Another 60 percent had Medicaid. The patient population served is virtually 100 percent black and Latino. If a white person happens to be hit by a car down the street from Sinai, then they might be brought there. Otherwise a white patient, or anyone who is well insured, would rarely set foot inside Sinai.

Then there's Northwestern Memorial Hospital. One of the top hospitals in the United States, on the *US News and World Report* Honor Roll, it towers over Lake Michigan about five miles from Sinai, in Chicago's predominantly white Streeterville neighborhood. It has an A bond rating, and about 500 days of cash brimming in its accounts. This translates to $2 billion in bank reserves. Most of Northwestern's largely white patient population has private insurance. A small number are uninsured.

During my time at Sinai, there were often only a few days of cash on hand. Sinai had no bond rating—meaning no bank would lend it money for capital investments. Just as Lawndale had been redlined seventy years prior, Sinai and other hospitals that serve poor communities are redlined by the banking industry today, limited in their ability to borrow. Sinai has been an anchor in the Lawndale neighborhood since 1919, and it takes care of everyone who comes to its doors, regardless of ability to pay. The price of this noble mission is a hospital's equivalent to a vow of poverty. From a banker's perspective Sinai is a bad investment.

Compare Northwestern and Mount Sinai's spending on capital in 2012. Capital dollars reflect the amount of money that a hospital has to spend on patients, doctors, equipment, and upgrades. Northwestern spent $273 million on buildings and equipment. Sinai spent just $6 million.[46] The failure of capital markets to support Sinai contributed to its chronic struggles to maintain service quality. If we really want to achieve equity in health care outcomes, then we have to invest more into the institutions serving those who need care the most, like Sinai. This means redistributing capital dollars based on need from Northwestern and its neighborhoods to invest in Sinai and its Lawndale neighborhood. This is just the opposite of how the American health care system works. In America we have arranged it so those who need it the most (often black people and other minorities) get less, while those with the most (white and affluent people) get the best care and facilities available in the world. It is no surprise that life expectancy in Northwestern's neighborhood is 85 years. In Sinai's neighborhood it is 72 years.[47]

Failure to Rescue

When it comes to providing the highest quality of care, volume matters. The doctors and the nursing staff who are exposed to high volumes of particular kinds of cases have more time to hone their skills, and this leads to better outcomes. A surgeon who does liver transplants every week is better at them than one who does one per year. As for complex surgical conditions where high volumes of cases are crucial to achieve the best outcomes, nonwhite patients are more likely than whites to receive them at low-volume institutions. These patients are also less likely to be rescued if they deteriorate postoperatively. Procedural complication rates are exactly the same at high-mortality and low-mortality hospitals. So what is the reason for the death gap? The answer is called *failure to rescue*. When a sick patient gets a complication, the doctors and nurses have to recognize and treat it—that is, rescue the patient from dying. Hospitals with well-developed systems to recognize complications and rescue patients have lower mortality.[48] While all the components of rescue have not been identified, adequate nurse staffing and training is critical. The hospitals with the least capability to rescue—due to nursing shortages, lack of training opportunities for staff, or other factors—serve significantly more minority patients and suffer higher mortality rates.[49]

Truth or Consequences

Cardiac surgery at Mount Sinai Hospital is an example of a low-volume and high-mortality program. Its struggles are instructive for understanding the day-to-day decisions in a poor hospital and how they lead to health inequities. When I worked there, the heart surgery program was small—about fifty cases each year. Programs this small have trouble maintaining quality because there is not enough repetition for all the staff who need to be in top form. In addition, because the capital investments required to maintain the service were so high, Sinai managers thought the limited capital we had should be invested elsewhere. So we closed the program and partnered with a nearby, higher-volume academic medical center (University of Illinois) to take our patients. It made sense. The neighborhood did not need a small, poorly functioning heart-surgery program.

Then one day we had a patient in the cardiac-care unit with three blocked coronary arteries. He needed emergency bypass surgery. Our cardiologists inserted a special pump into his aorta to boost to his failing heart until lifesaving cardiac surgery could be performed. Time was critical. But the patient was uninsured, and the University of Illinois refused the patient. In desperation I phoned the chief of cardiology there. He recommended that the patient be discharged from Sinai and instructed to walk into the University of Illinois emergency room. Then, he said they would be required to treat him. I was shocked. Not only was this immoral, but it was medical malpractice. The patient was hooked to life support, teetering on the edge of death with an artificial heart pump attached to a blood vessel in his groin. Without surgery soon he would surely die. It took a call from our CEO to U of I's CEO to get this patient transferred.

After this event, against their better judgment, our cardiologists urged our CEO to restart cardiac surgery at Mount Sinai. Despite the low volumes, inability to guarantee quality, and high capital costs, it became a necessary investment. These are the choices faced by safety-net hospitals in communities of concentrated disadvantage. Provide nothing and let patients die from neglect; or provide the best care you can, at risk of higher than desired mortality, and hope to pull most patients through.

More broadly, a 2014 study evaluated cardiac-surgery mortality in patients insured by Medicare. Nonwhite patients succumbed at a 33 percent higher rate than whites (after risk factors were controlled for). Thirty-five percent of the death gap was due to deficiencies in hospital quality. The highest-mortality hospitals were those that served predominantly minority populations. Both white and black patients who received their heart surgery at predominantly minority hospitals had higher mortality rates, suggesting structural factors were responsible.

When we speak of institutionalized racism as a structural cause of premature death, it is not the virulent type of racism that we associate with opposition to the civil rights movement of the 1960s. It's a more banal but deadly form of brutality woven into the tapestries of our institutions and thus harder to eradicate. I was not shocked by the study's findings.[50] I knew that race itself—as a social marker—was not the reason for the cardiac mortality gap at predominantly minority hospitals; it was our tolerance for inequality in quality across our health care system. This becomes even more obvious when we contrast these findings with the outcomes in the Veterans Administration system, where care is structured the same way nationwide. In the VA system there is no equivalent racial heart-disease death gap.[51]

Inequality in Quality and Unequal Treatment

It is not only in majority minority hospitals that black health-care inequities exist. When black and brown patients receive medical care in any setting, they are more likely than white patients to receive unequal care. This was documented in the Institute of Medicine's shocking *Unequal Treatment* report, which synthesized hundreds of studies of age, sex, and racial differences in medical diagnoses, treatments, and health care outcomes. The report concluded that for almost every disease studied, black Americans received less effective care than white Americans. These disparities prevailed even among groups with identical socioeconomic or insurance status. Minority patients received fewer recommended treatments for diseases ranging from AIDS to cancer to heart disease.[52] How much of the treatment gap is related to implicit bias, patient mistrust, physician practice style, or systematic organizational dysfunction is not known, but these gaps have persisted over the decade and more since the Institute of Medicine report.[53] Each year since 2003, the Agency for Health Care Quality and Research has tracked progress on health care inequity across America, analyzing more than 250 quality measures across a broad array of settings and services. In the 2014 report, the agency reported no overall improvement in racial health disparities from prior years. Not one iota.

The American Hospital Association Pledge

In 2015, in response to years of intractable health care inequities, the American Hospital Association called upon CEOs of hospitals across America to sign a pledge to measure health inequities within their own institutions and to fix them. The Equity of Care Campaign to End Healthcare Disparities focus is on four areas. First, hospitals are to choose a quality measure that is important to their community. Next, they are to develop a plan to address a disparity, whether by race, ethnicity, or language preference. Third, hospitals are asked to provide cultural competency training for all staff or finalize a plan to do so. Finally, hospital operations teams are asked to initiate a dialogue with the board and leadership team about this disparity work.[54]

After over a century of documented health-care disparities, this step is important. But it is hardly enough. The nation's hospitals have been organized for the most part to make money by attracting the best clientele with the best insurance policies. For most hospitals this means avoiding poor and minority neighborhoods. Those frayed and capital-poor hospitals that have made it their mission to care for poor and uninsured often struggle in poverty like their clients.

Just as the neighborhoods of concentrated disadvantage were created by white and industrial flight and the expansion of neighborhoods of concentrated advantage, a similar phenomenon has occurred in health care. The nation's wealthiest health care systems for the most part have

avoided serving the residents of concentrated disadvantage by placing offices and hospitals only in white communities of advantage. So
pledges are well and good, but without larger structural changes that
level the insurance and capital decisions that underpin the health care
system, health care equity will continue to be elusive.

Only with national health insurance reform that begins with the
idea of health as a human right could these structural issues be re-
solved. The Affordable Care Act, the most recent response to the need
for health care reform, has tried to address these issues. However, as
we will see, it has been an inadequate solution so far.

THE POISON PILL

HEALTH INSURANCE IN AMERICA

You guys are evil. Canada's the best country in the world. We go to the doctor and we don't have to worry about paying him, but here your whole life you're broke because of medical bills.[1]

JUSTIN BIEBER

It will not do to note that under the Affordable Care Act almost 90 percent of Americans currently have some form of health insurance, any more than it would do for a hotel to note that 90 percent of the time the roof over your bed does not leak when it rains.[2] Of all possible ways to remedy structural violence in America, the creation of an equitable universal health-care system based on the idea that health care is a right, not a commodity, ranks high. While the health care law was a reform of the old system that saw fifty million Americans uninsured, the Affordable Care Act perpetuates health care inequity and fragmentation by its very design. Yet if Republican calls to repeal the law are heeded, we will be back to square one. And bad will revert to worse.

I was not surprised that the solution for universal health care in the United States would be to prop up the existing costly, inequitable, and inefficient insurance system. In 2003 my wife and I cosponsored a fundraiser in Chicago for the then little-known Illinois state senator Barack Obama, who was running for the US Senate. In the living room of a modest single-family home in the neatly manicured South Shore neighborhood of Chicago, I asked the future president his position on national health-care reform. His words presaged what came to be known as "Obamacare."

"I'm a proponent of a single-payer system," he responded. But he explained that the political power held by the health insurance companies was so formidable that opposing them would be political suicide. He noted that the insurance industry had over 250,000 employees across the country and a lobbying apparatus that had to be reckoned with in any drive for universal health care. "Single payer will never get passed in the United States," he concluded.

He was correct. Single payer did not even get a hearing. The Affordable Care Act was a modest reform of the existing tiered health-insurance system, which treats health care as a commodity, not a human right. The coverage provisions in the Affordable Care Act built on and attempted to fill in the gaps in a piecemeal system that had left many without affordable coverage.

There have not been impressive gains since the passage of health reform.[3] A net of twenty million more people gained health insurance coverage between 2013 and 2015. Medicaid has expanded in thirty-two states and the District of Columbia, providing new access to coverage to millions of previously uninsurable Americans.[4] The Affordable Care Act has been successful in reducing the number of uninsured, but about 30 million Americans remain uninsured.[5] Most important, the Affordable Care Act fails two critical parameters of health justice: it is neither universal nor equitable.

Elegant, Equitable, and Not to Be

The most elegant, comprehensive, fairest, and lowest-cost solution to the health care crisis would have been to expand and improve the Medicare insurance plan to cover all Americans.[6] Medicare, enacted in 1965 as a single governmental payer system to provide health insurance for Americans 65 and older, has been well liked since its inception. Before Medicare, 48 percent of such Americans had no insurance; now only 2 percent are uninsured. In addition, before Medicare 56 percent of senior Americans paid out-of-pocket health care expenses, compared to 13 percent now.[7] Satisfaction with coverage is substantially higher among Medicare recipients than for those who have private insurance. Only 8 percent of Medicare enrollees report their experience as fair or poor, compared to 20 percent of those with typical employer-based health insurance coverage and 33 percent of those who purchased private insurance directly.[8] Moreover, the costs of administering the program are substantially lower than those of private insurance companies—only about 2 percent of the total cost for Medicare, compared to 12 percent for the least expensive insurance company's overhead charges.[9] Most important, experts estimate that since its inception Medicare has added five years to the life expectancy of older Americans.[10] Polls have shown that universal government-sponsored health coverage is preferred by half of Americans.[11] And an improved Medicare would be an entitlement available to all Americans, with the exact same benefits for the wealthy and the poor. Medicare for all would achieve the goal of universal access to health care. As an entitlement for all US citizens (and extended to noncitizen residents), access to health care would be a right. This would contribute to the improvement of the life expectancy gap between rich and poor. Plus it would save an estimated $400 billion yearly by eliminating administrative waste.[12]

So if one wanted to solve the problem of the uninsured and reduce the death gaps between rich and poor, expansion of Medicare with other enhancements would have been the most logical approach. This is not a radical idea. Thirty advanced industrialized nations have forms of universal health care.[13] Canada has a "Medicare for All" health insurance with easier access to care, lower costs, and better health outcomes (including life expectancy) than those of the United States. The evidence is compelling. While health inequity has not been eliminated in Canada, the differences between poor and rich are not as striking as they are in the United States.[14] In Canada, men in the poorest urban neighborhoods experienced the biggest declines in mortality from heart disease from 1971 to 1996.[15] Life expectancy gaps between income groups declined during that period as well. Poor Canadians with cancer had better survival than poor people from Detroit, an outcome attributed to the Canadian system.[16] Of all the major Western economic powers, the United States is the only one without a universal health care system in which health care is considered a human right.[17]

Rather than treating access to health insurance as a universal right, the language of the Affordable Care Act endorsed the idea that health care is a mandate.[18] The difference between health care as a right and health care as a mandate is critical, as these conceptions lead to very divergent solutions. If health care is a right, universal health care is an entitlement that should be the same for all citizens. If health care is a mandate, however, then there is no such entitlement, and health care is a commodity to be bought and sold. The Affordable Care Act established the mandate as a core component of health care coverage, perpetuating the complex system of multiple payers, limited access, variability in quality of care, high costs, and large rich-poor life expectancy gaps.

Obamacare and Beyond

The 2010 Affordable Care Act remains the most significant overhaul of the American health care system since the passage of Medicare in 1965, expanding insurance coverage to millions. The law survived multiple attempts by Congress and two Supreme Court challenges that aimed to gut its major provisions.[19] As a reform of the current for-profit insurance marketplace, the Affordable Care Act addressed two major gaps in the existing system. First, it allowed young adults to stay on their parents' health insurance until the age of twenty-six—a popular provision that benefits almost eight million Americans.[20] The second major reform prevented insurers from denying coverage to people with preexisting medical conditions. Medicaid was expanded to include millions of previously uninsurable individuals who had been excluded from the health care system. Uninsured rates among whites, blacks, and Hispanics dropped, narrowing though not eliminating racial and ethnic insurance coverage gaps.[21]

At the same time, the Affordable Care Act incorporated the worst aspects of our fragmented for-profit health insurance system. The tiered system of insurance—where the coverage options for the poor are markedly different from those for the rich—has further hardwired inequity into the law.

In 2004 there were fifty million people without health insurance in the United States. That year the Institute of Medicine published a report, "Insuring America's Health," that outlined the principles against which any health reform legislation would have to be measured.[22] The institute identified the ideal system as having "universal, continuous insurance coverage that is affordable and sustainable for individuals, families, and society, and should enhance well-being through care that is effective, efficient, safe, timely, patient-centered, and equitable." Eleven years later, none of these standards was being met. Even after the passage of the Affordable Care Act, there are around thirty million Americans without insurance and an equal number of underinsured who have health insurance policies but with deductibles and copayments that are high enough to deter care.[23]

How did the United States end up with a more fragmented, more costly, and more confusing health care system? Simply stated, collusion between members of Congress and entrenched corporate health insurance and Big Pharma interests precluded a more equitable and lower-cost solution. What Americans got with the Affordable Care Act was complicated insurance marketplaces in every state with a complex array of confusing private insurance products. The health reform process exposed, in the words of the British medical journal *The Lancet*, "how corporate influence renders the US Government incapable of making policy on the basis of evidence and the public interest."[24] When the moment arrived to consider having a Medicare-like "public option" on the state exchanges to compete with private insurance companies, Senator Joseph Lieberman of Connecticut, the deciding Senate vote, deep-sixed the idea by threatening a filibuster.[25] The capital of Connecticut is Hartford, the home of Aetna, one of the big five health insurance companies.

Skin in the Game

There are three major structural flaws in the Affordable Care Act, all of which could be solved by a single-payer system. The first flaw is that the insurance expansion is neither universal nor equitable. For example, because mandatory Medicaid expansion was blocked by the Supreme Court, nineteen states have left millions of poor people uninsured.[26] These states account for over half of poor uninsured blacks, single mothers, and the country's uninsured working poor. For poor people in these states, it is as if Obamacare was never enacted. Note that for the most part these states that have refused to expand Medicaid are the former Confederate slaveholding states, accentuating the legacy of structural racism. Access to specialty care for those who receive Medicaid coverage is limited compared to access for patients with private insurance.[27] More than one-third of US doctors refuse to take Medicaid—another structural barrier.[28]

The second flaw is that premiums, copays, and deductibles for private health insurance and products on the marketplaces are prohibitively high for many people, especially the working poor. In 2015 average annual premiums for employer-sponsored health insurance were $6,251 for single coverage and $17,545 for family coverage. Between 2014 and 2015, premiums increased by 4 percent, while during the same period workers' wages increased 1.9 percent. Premiums for family coverage increased 27 percent during the last five years, while cost sharing has skyrocketed.[29] The average individual deductible across the marketplace plans in 2016 was $5,765 for bronze plans. After the deductible is paid, an individual with such a plan will face 40 percent copays for services.[30] Insurance companies have reacted to their rising costs by creating narrow networks of providers and hospitals.[31] This limits choice of patients by restricting the doctors and hospitals whose services they can use.

At the heart of the Affordable Care Act are subsidies for the working poor to pay for health insurance premiums.[32] The goal was to keep these premiums within reach of most Americans. It was a sweet deal for the insurance companies. The insurance companies are guaranteed to get their premiums; the federal government poured billions of dollars into their coffers. In exchange, an individual gets an insurance card. But with that card came unprecedented out-of-pocket expenses that kicked in before the insurance company paid one cent.[33] The belief is that without "skin in the game," the newly insured will overuse the system. As a result, coinsurance and deductibles that many Americans now are forced to pay have skyrocketed across the insurance markets. Yet every study ever done on the impact of copays and deductibles (even for middle-class people) is that they cause individuals to delay medical care.[34] Under a single-payer health care system there would be no copays or deductibles.

Obamacare Bullshit

The third flaw of the Affordable Care Act was that long-term doctor-patient relationships have been disrupted by insurance restrictions. President Obama said, "No matter how we reform health care, I intend to keep this promise: If you like your doctor, you'll be able to keep your doctor; if you like your health care plan, you'll be able to keep your health care plan."[35] This turned out to be untrue.

Windora Bradley, a year before her stroke, struggled to pay her health insurance premiums. Faced with the dilemma to buy food or go without medications, she chose to go without medications. At one of her office visits, she let loose.

"I'm tired about this Obamacare bullshit," she shook her head, frowning as her jowls quivered. "I worked for thirty-five years. Those people on welfare who never worked are getting free health care. I am paying $700 each month and there is not enough left for medicines and food. That's not right. That's why I call it Obamacare bullshit."

Windora lived on a pension of about $1,000 per month. Most went for the premiums on her health insurance, which she still received through the Chicago Board of Education. She scrimped and saved to pay for her medications for her diabetes, hypertension, asthma, and vascular disease. Her situation is common among the working poor.

Windora was ultimately able to get insurance on the marketplace that reduced her premium costs but not her out-of-pocket expenses. At first she purchased a Blue Cross insurance plan that she was told my hospital accepted, but this proved incorrect. She then had to purchase a more expensive plan to stay with me. Meanwhile her two sisters, who had also been my patients for over thirty years, had to switch doctors because my group did not accept the insurance they enrolled in. A number of my long-term patients found themselves in this dilemma. In 2015, after her stroke, Blue Cross dropped my hospital and many others from the plan Windora had just purchased. There was only one plan, from United Health Care, in all of Cook County that included my hospital and me in the network. The week after Windora signed up for it, United Health Care let it be known that it was considering withdrawing from all the exchanges in 2017.[36]

In three years of the Affordable Care Act, Windora had purchased three different insurance policies just to retain me as her physician. In the fall of 2016, United Health Care announced it would drop my hospital from its network, and Windora, now wheelchair bound and speechless, is forced to find another doctor (to say nothing of her many specialitsts) after thirty-six years. For someone like Windora with complex medical and social obstacles, keeping a team of providerss who are familiar with her medical travails is essential to getting good care. For me, her longtime doctor, it is a gut-wrenching experience.

The fact is that Obamacare, despite its modest benefits, does not remedy American health care inequity. It will never achieve universal coverage. Eleven million noncitizen residents will never be eligible for its benefits. Thirty million people will remain uninsured. While insurance coverage has increased for all races, there is still a large racial and ethnic gap in insurance coverage, which will perpetuate health disparities. For those with health insurance, spiraling copays and deductibles have made access to care more difficult. Finally, by allowing a dizzying array of for-profit insurance carriers with high administrative overhead expenses, the Affordable Care Act as currently configured will not control costs.

In 2016, the third year of Obamacare, insurance companies asked for double-digit increases in premium prices, as they claimed costs of delivery had outstripped the revenues. Meanwhile, health insurance stocks are trading at all-time highs, while patients like Windora Bradley face rocketing expenses and uncertainty about the future.[37]

A Call for Single Payer

I speak for many of my health care colleagues across the nation when I say that the Affordable Care Act is a disappointment. In contrast, an improved and expanded Medicare for All would achieve truly universal care, affordability, equity, and effective cost control. It would put the interests of our patients—and our nation's health—first. By replacing multiple private insurers with a single nonprofit agency like Medicare that pays all medical bills, the United States would save approximately $400 billion annually. Administrative bloat in our current private-insurance-based system would be slashed. That waste would be redirected to clinical care. Copays, coinsurance, and deductibles would be eliminated. A single streamlined system would be able to rein in costs for medications and other supplies through the system's strong bargaining clout—clout directed to benefit health, not profits. Finally, it would create an equitable system of care that would provide equal access to rich, poor, black, and white. As a result, life expectancy gaps between rich and poor would narrow. Hospitals that serve poor communities would have access to capital investment based on need. It has been done in other countries, and it can be done in the United States.

Single-payer health care stands in stark contrast to the ACA's incremental reform. Yet it is important to remember that enactment of a single-payer system requires the defeat of deeply vested, deep-pocketed ideological opponents, health insurance conglomerates, and a thick alliance of health care constituencies along with other interest groups. The Affordable Care Act, passed by a Democratic majority and signed by a Democratic president, was a weak compromise that left the foundations of our flawed $2.9 trillion health care system intact. It will be some time before political conditions are again right to tackle an improved Medicare for All. So why, given these hurdles, do I (and many other health care providers) persist? I persist because I have watched too many patients suffer and die because they lacked health insurance or had the wrong insurance card. I persist because I have witnessed the racial and ethnic death gaps enabled by our current health insurance arrangements. I persist because simple fairness dictates that health care is a fundamental human right. I persist because of patients like Windora and Sarai, who deserve better. For those who counter that single payer is too expensive or politically unfeasible, we persist because the American ideal of "life and liberty" cannot be achieved without an equitable and universal health care system.

Winston Churchill reportedly said, "You can always count on the Americans to do the right thing… after they have tried everything else."[38] We have tried everything else. I look forward to being part of a single-payer health care system that values the health of individuals, families, and communities as a common good—where health care is valued as a human right. Someday.

PART 4
THE CURE

11

COMMUNITY EFFICACY AND THE DEATH GAP

With segregation, with the isolation of the injured and the robbed, comes the concentration of disadvantage. An unsegregated America might see poverty, and all its effects, spread across the country with no particular bias toward skin color. Instead, the concentration of poverty has been paired with a concentration of melanin.[1]

TA-NEHISI COATES

It is now all too clear that public policies, social inequities, and health-care system factors are causing death gaps across the country. We know that neighborhoods of concentrated poverty and segregation promote ill health and early death. But are there communities that have resisted the cycle of structural violence and achieved better health outcomes and longer life expectancy? We know what makes a neighborhood sick. But do we know what makes a community healthy? Can the social and civic life in a community lift community health? Three distinct Chicago-area neighborhoods with vastly different mortality experiences—Chatham, Roseland, and west suburban Oak Park—can help us explore this question.

The Murder of Officer Thomas Wortham

This story begins with a tragedy. On May 19, 2010, Officer Thomas Wortham IV, police officer and Iraq War veteran, was shot and killed in front of his parents' house in the Chatham neighborhood on Chicago's South Side.[2] As Wortham left his parents' home, he had encountered four young men trying to steal his motorcycle. One of them pulled a gun and shot Wortham point blank.[3] Wortham collapsed to the ground, bleeding from an upper abdominal wound, and died an hour later.

The attack, and the confusion that surrounded it, disrupted many of Chatham residents' perception of their neighborhood. Chatham is a neighborhood of brick bungalows, manicured lawns, and well-kept apartment buildings. Families have lived there for generations. The schools were, by city standards, good. Crime was low. Community leaders were obsessive about maintaining the middle-class character of the neighborhood, and community organizations such as baseball leagues were abundant and filled with volunteer coaches. Wortham himself had been active in the community and served as president of the Nat King Cole Park Advisory Council.

Chatham had a reputation as a community where neighbor looked after neighbor and defended the character of the neighborhood. It had long had an active and engaged community, even while surrounding neighborhoods were destabilized by high levels of unemployment and poverty. The African American population of Chatham, originally a white middle-class neighborhood, had grown from 1 percent in 1950 to 97 percent in 2009.[4] Unlike most Chicago neighborhoods in which this racial transition occurred, Chatham remained a middle-class community, perhaps the only such neighborhood in the city to do so—and perhaps the only South Side neighborhood that could reasonably be said to have *improved* after white flight. Throughout the 1980s and 1990s, Chatham had a strong local economy and housing was in demand.[5] There were relatively few apartment, retail, or office vacancies.

But Chatham had fallen onto rough times since the 2007 recession. The neighborhood's confidence, if not its resolve, was shaken. Housing prices had plummeted. Many homeowners had foreclosed, and boarded-up houses, never before seen there, dotted the streets. Unemployment was up. New residents, some from recently torn-down public housing high-rises a few miles away, had moved into the close-knit neighborhood. Street violence—armed robberies and murder—

had increased. Because of a recent rash of shootings, the alderman had removed the basketball hoops in Cole Park.

Just the week before his murder, Wortham, a third-generation resident of Chatham, had spoken to the *Chicago Tribune* about the violence in his neighborhood. "It's starting to feel like it's expected in this community," he said. "When people think of the South Side of Chicago, they think violence. In Chatham, that's not what we see. It's happened, and we're going to fix it, so it doesn't happen again."[6]

Like Chatham, neighboring Roseland has a population that consists of mainly non-Hispanic black residents. Even though the difference in annual per capita income between Chatham and Roseland between 2008 and 2012 was just $932, the poverty rate in Chatham was actually higher than that in Roseland. Yet despite the poverty rate and its recent stresses, Chatham has consistently demonstrated better health outcomes than comparable neighborhoods. According to a city report in 2013, Chatham scored better in stroke, cancer, and diabetes death rates and had a higher life expectancy when compared to Roseland.[7]

In what ways does Chatham differ from Roseland that would explain these variations? The communities are adjacent and face similar structural obstacles of racism and poverty. Is there some other insulating force that helps to support Chatham's residents and protect their health, which Roseland lacks?

The answer may lie in the community itself. When compared to all neighborhoods in Chicago, Chatham's level of social cohesion ranks second after that of Avalon Park, a community with a similar racial composition but a higher per capita income.[8] Social cohesion can be defined as the connectedness between neighbors. For example, do people in a community trust one another, or is there a deep level of cynicism and distrust? Another key factor here is efficacy. Self-efficacy is the ability of a person to navigate through life. People who have a sense of purpose in life have greater self-efficacy. Social cohesion is the trusting interconnectedness among a group of neighbors. It is an essential element of collective efficacy (or collective purpose), which is social cohesion plus the willingness of a group of neighbors to act together for the common good.[9]

Social cohesion and collective efficacy might explain why Chatham's life expectancy is higher than Roseland's. Cohesion alone cannot over-come the downward spiral of health that poverty and its associated ills can create in a neighborhood. But social cohesion and collective efficacy might have mitigating impacts on the deleterious health effects of poverty. Social cohesion enables neighbors to take action. That is what happened in Chatham. Wortham's death rekindled neighbor-hood action. The day after his killing, community members and local police officers assembled at Cole Park to "take back the park," a place that had once been a central part of social life for many young families. Since then, some Chatham residents have started a fund to buy fore-closed homes and resell them to "people who will make good neigh-bors."[10] Nevertheless, the bounceback from the economic decline in the late 2000s was sluggish; the 2007–11 American Community Survey found that 25.2 percent of Chatham households were below the pov-erty line.[11]

Chatham is not the only community where engaged neighbors have contributed to the health of their community. Take Oak Park (life ex-pectancy 81), a suburb that shares a more-than-three-mile border with the impoverished Austin neighborhood on the west side of Chicago (life expectancy 72). Oak Park used citizen action and public policy to achieve successful long-term racial integration and good health.

The Oak Park Model

I have lived in Oak Park since the mid-1980s. With its tree-lined streets and parks with soccer fields and basketball courts, it looks like a healthy community. The birthplace of Ernest Hemingway and the site of many Frank Lloyd Wright–designed homes, Oak Park is a cultural touchstone in the Chicago area. In 1964, residents of the then all-white community, faced with the specter of blockbusting, panic peddling, and rapid white flight in Austin just to the east, took matters into their own hands: They welcomed black residents to town by adopting public policies that aimed to ease white fears about having black neighbors. Given white attitudes about blacks, it was not a surprise that many were skeptical that Oak Park could avoid the rapid housing and community turmoil experienced by every neighborhood on Chicago's West Side.

But social cohesion and community efficacy allowed the community to manage to achieve racial integration and maintain low mortality rates.

One key step was the difficult and emotional passage of a fair housing ordinance, years before the federal Fair Housing Act of 1968.[12] Proponents faced death threats. Fear of rapid and destabilizing racial turnover gripped the village. But a group of community activists believed that Oak Park could successfully become a racially integrated village.[13] The Fair Housing ordinance created a Community Relations Commission with the mandate of addressing whites' fears of integration. Once the ordinance was passed, the police chief of Oak Park and other village officials visited white homeowners to convince them to welcome future African American neighbors and to squelch rumors that might fuel white flight. One result, a half-century later, is that 81% percent of Oak Park blocks have at least one black family, there are no segregated apartment buildings, and there are no segregated census tracts.[14] This is a feat considering the hypersegregation in neighboring Chicago; Austin is 97 percent black, while Edison Park has a population that is 93.6 percent white.[15]

However, the fair housing ordinance and the work of the Community Relations Commission would have accomplished little if not for focused measures taken to prevent the predatory real estate practices that plagued many neighborhoods of Chicago.[16] Along Madison Street in the Austin neighborhood in the five years prior to the passing of the fair housing ordinance, eighteen blocks flipped from all white to all black.[17] Urbanologist Pierre DeVise predicted that Oak Park would be hit next with rapid neighborhood change.[18] Having witnessed blockbusting tactics and the destabilizing effects that the rapid racial transition had on surrounding communities, a group of Oak Park residents proposed that the village establish a housing action center to oversee the integration of the housing market. The Oak Park Housing Center was started as a volunteer effort in a second-floor room of the First Congregational Church.

Unlike the Community Relations Commission, the housing center took direct action against the blockbusting practices of the speculators. One of the center's programs retrained real estate agents to prevent racial steering (the practice of showing houses and apartments to black people only in black neighborhoods) and to sell the diversity of the community as a positive, not a negative. As a result, the realty community in Oak Park, on the whole, never engaged in racial steering.[19] The housing center also put ads in liberal magazines like *Harper's* and *The New Republic* to encourage whites who might embrace an integrated community to move to Oak Park to replace those fleeing from fear.[20]

Many of the policies implemented by the center were controversial (some thought coercive and proscriptive) but effective. It worked with apartment owners to spruce up their buildings and to enhance security. The center's leaders persuaded the Oak Park Housing Authority to buy and rehab deteriorating apartment buildings on the east side of town, near Austin. They persuaded the village to pass an "equity assurance" law to guarantee the selling price of homes and thus deter panic selling by whites.[21] With the consent of the local realtors, the center instituted a ban on "for sale" signs that still stands today. This was a further effort to mitigate against mass white flight and panic.[22] While such a ban is unconstitutional, no Oak Park homeowner has ever challenged it. A ban on overnight street parking and the creation of cul-de-sacs on the east end of the town gave the tree-lined streets and manicured lawns a reassuring, sedate, suburban appearance, especially in comparison to the urban squalor a few blocks to the east in Chicago. This also effectively sealed Oak Park from easy foot or car traffic from Austin. The town was accused of pandering to white fears, but addressing the racial dreads of whites was one of many strategies that led to Oak Park's racial integration. Oak Park remains a fairly diverse and integrated community, with a population that in 2010 was 63.8 percent non-Hispanic/Latino white, 31.7 percent black, 6.8 percent Hispanic/Latino, and 4.8 percent Asian.[23]

The success of Oak Park has been as much about changing the biases and perceptions of white and middle-class renters as it has been about fair housing. An earlier chapter of this book discussed how the presence of blacks or immigrants in a neighborhood triggered white perceptions of deteriorating quality.[24] Other studies on perception have found that whites tend to rate an affluent neighborhood with white residents much more highly than the same affluent neighborhood with blacks in it. It's not the neighborhood affluence that triggers the response, it is the race of the neighbors.[25] These experiments explain why Oak Park housing efforts focused on influencing white perceptions and biases.

Most of the neighborhood preference shaping took the form of steering potential white homeowners and renters to consider the east side of the village. This practice was considered "positive steering." Homebuyers and renters who seek assistance from the housing center are prompted to look at properties in an area with a lower concentration of people of their own race.[26] Positive steering aims to make sure that no area of the community has a high concentration of one racial or ethnic group.

Bobbie Raymond, the founder of the housing center, responded swiftly when the center was accused of steering and racism: "What we do is not steering. Steering is blacks who go looking for housing being escorted to black areas or integrated areas, and whites who look for housing being escorted to white areas, period. That's a very negative term, and I don't like for us to be lumped in with groups that steer. Our counseling and escorting is affirmative escorting, exposing whites and blacks to units they couldn't see otherwise. When we talk about 'integration maintenance,' we're really talking about trying to undo years of segregation maintenance."[27]

"If we weren't doing this work, Oak Park would probably remain diverse, but it would start segregating very quickly," says Rob Breymaier, the center's current executive director. Blacks are slightly overrepresented in Oak Park relative to the region. And they are not all clustered on the east side. Given how quickly rental units turn over, Breymaier estimates that without the center's efforts it would take only about five years for the village to become racially segregated. "This is not something we can stop doing," he says. "Unless there's an intention to promote integration, segregation often just happens because of the way our society is built."[28]

A key factor in the efforts to maintain an integrated community has been the involvement of the community itself: white community members adjusted to the incoming black residents in a way rarely seen in Chicago in the 1970s. This social cohesion has carried forward into the current day, cropping up in groups such as the Oak Park–River

Forest Community Foundation and the continuing work of the Oak Park Housing Center.[29] In fact, Oak Park was able to weather the economic recession of the early 2000s better than other areas in the region; 8.6 percent of its residents were under the poverty level for 2009–13, compared to a rate of 14.1 percent in the city of Chicago.[30]

Collective Efficacy, Social Capital, and Health

Chatham and Oak Park have a common characteristic of community involvement and social cohesion. However, it is clear that the ability of these two places to bounce back from the Great Recession varied greatly. Moreover, the health outcomes of these two communities are worlds apart. The age-adjusted death rate in Oak Park was 698.0 per 100,000 persons from 2006 to 2008.[31] During a similar period (2007–9) in Chatham, the age-adjusted death rate was 905.3 per 100,000 persons.[32] Though Chatham's health outcomes were better than Roseland's, both of these neighborhoods lagged behind Oak Park. The death rates from cancer, diabetes, and stroke are all lower in Oak Park than in both Roseland and Chatham.

As with Oak Park's transformation from a predominantly white town to a diverse and integrated area or Chatham's fierce protection of its neighborhood character, communities can manage social change and preserve health—but some neighborhoods are better able to do so than others. One way to understand the level of cohesion and the strength of social forces in a community is through the concept of collective efficacy. This concept was explored in the Project on Human Development in Chicago Neighborhoods (PHDCN) in the late 1990s.[33] Drawing on this project, which he ran, in his 2012 book *Great American City*, Robert J. Sampson defines collective efficacy as "the linkage of cohesion and mutual trust among residents with shared expectations for intervening in support of neighborhood social control."[34]

In the PHDCN, researchers measured the amount of collective efficacy in Chicago's neighborhoods through the use of surveys that asked questions such as "If a group of neighborhood children were skipping school and hanging out on a street corner, how likely is it that your neighbors would do something about it?" and "If there was a fight in

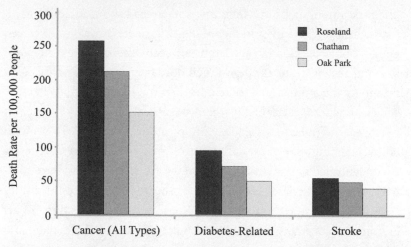

Neighborhoods with high degrees of social cohesion and community efficacy have lower rates of mortality from cancer, diabetes, and stroke. Roseland and Chatham are black communities with similar levels of poverty. Chatham, however, has much higher levels of community efficacy and cohesion. Its mortality rates are lower than Roseland's. Oak Park is a mixed-race suburban community with about one-third the poverty level of Chatham and Roseland. It has even lower mortality rates. Source: Chicago Department of Public Health and Robert Sampson, *The Great American City*.

front of your house... how likely is it that your neighbors would break it up?"[35] After reviewing these data, researchers were able to classify neighborhoods by level of collective efficacy. Essentially, in neighborhoods such as Chatham, where they found high levels of collective efficacy, community members were more likely to speak up if they saw something suspect, and they felt that their neighbors were likely to do the same.[36]

A second, related way to observe the level of social cohesion and the significance of community in an area is to look at social capital. There are varying understandings of social capital, but it is often defined as "[the] features of social structure—such as trust, norms, and networks—that facilitate collective action for mutual benefit."[37] Thus, unlike collective efficacy, which takes into account only the actions taken by members of the community, social capital traces the broader social pathways and arrangements that allow for collective action.

Chatham and Oak Park are communities with high social capital.

The link among collective efficacy, social capital, place, and health makes sense: if one lives in an area with grocery stores, safe streets, good schools, parks, and access to health care, there is a better chance of living a healthy life. But how much does the geography of the community make a difference to health? Can the community itself—the social networks, relationships, and organizations—improve health outcomes? Both factors are likely important. Communities with high efficacy and high social capital that are surrounded by neighborhoods of concentrated poverty and disadvantage are more likely to have spillovers of poverty-related crime and poor health than are communities surrounded by other high-efficacy communities. Perhaps this in part explains the mortality gap between Chatham and Oak Park. Oak Park, while bordering hypersegregated Austin on its east, has wealthy River Forest to its west and gentrifying Berwyn to its south. Chatham on the other hand, is a middle-class island in a sea of concentrated and segregated poverty.

One of the more interesting associations is the relationship between community efficacy and life expectancy. Sampson found that communities with medium or high collective efficacy have a significantly greater life expectancy than communities with low collective efficacy.[38] In fact, the difference between the average life expectancies for communities with high and low collective efficacy was more than six years. In those "extra" six years, people who live in communities with high collective efficacy could watch their children graduate from college or see their grandchildren start first grade. The small difference of a few blocks and the level of social cohesion in a community can have a great impact on one's life arc.

Communities that are high in collective efficacy also exhibit a high degree of social altruism. In both Oak Park and Chatham there is a strong sense of "neighbor looking after neighbor" that is not as common in other neighborhoods. These neighborhoods have higher rates of "bystander CPR"—the chance that a stranger will initiate CPR on a random stranger who collapses on the street.[39] Not only may it feel good to live in a community with high levels of social cohesion and efficacy, it can greatly affect one's health—and the likelihood that one would survive a heart attack, a heat wave, or a bout of breast cancer.

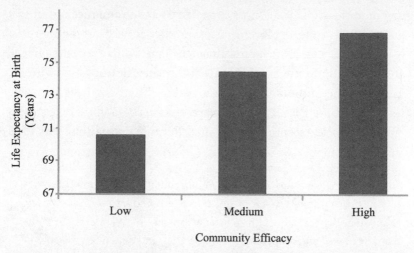

Neighborhoods that have higher social cohesion among members and higher measures of community effectiveness have higher life expectancies than those without. In neighborhoods with high collective efficacy, neighbors look out for each other, and community organizations are active in neighborhood betterment. This suggests that empowered communities are healthier communities. Source: Chicago Department of Public Health, Healthy Chicago Reports, 2014, and Robert Sampson, *Great American City*.

Rare Black Collective Efficacy

Yet even though the association of collective efficacy and mortality is powerful, another observation about collective efficacy brings pause. Sampson's work reveals that neighborhoods with medium or high collective efficacy had a significantly lower population of black residents than those with low collective efficacy.[40]

Inversely, neighborhoods with high collective efficacy had a larger white population in 2000 when compared to neighborhoods with low or medium collective efficacy.[41] The fact is, it is unusual for an all-black community to have high collective efficacy. So is it that white people just tend to have closer-knit communities, or is there something else, such as exploitation, concentrated poverty, and racism, that explains the efficacy gap?

In view of my earlier discussion of the disastrous effects of concentrated disadvantage, we should look at collective efficacy through the lens of privilege. Because Chicago is hypersegregated, there are communities in which almost all residents are of one racial or ethnic group, often white or black. If a community consists of a group that has historically faced structural violence in the form of social, political, and economic barriers, collective efficacy may not be able to thrive. Though some communities of color, such as Chatham, have been able to maintain their levels of collective efficacy through concentrated efforts, it is the exception rather than the rule. Explaining this idea, Sampson writes:

> Research has demonstrated that an individual's socioeconomic status is positively linked to his or her sense of personal control, efficacy, and even biological health. A similar process may work at the community level, where alienation, exploitation, and dependency wrought by resource deprivation act as a centrifugal force that stymies collective efficacy. Even if personal ties are strong in areas of concentrated disadvantage, they may be weakly tethered to collective actions.[42]

Socioeconomic status can affect not only an individual's health and feeling of well-being but also that of an entire community. If a neighborhood is faced with poverty and other structural obstacles, there may not be room for community development, even if neighbors are friendly and look out for one another. White communities have the privilege of taking part in activities that build collective efficacy and social capital because they do not face the multitude of roadblocks that impede many black and other poor communities.

Furthermore, it may be dangerous to point to collective efficacy and community development as a health improvement strategy, as it places the responsibility for health outcomes squarely on these disadvantaged communities. Such responsibility may provide a collective sense of agency and a way for disadvantaged communities to heal themselves, as in the case of Chatham. However, *enabling* communities to gain this agency and *expecting* them to take this responsibility are two very different propositions. An expectation that communities should take this responsibility allows blame to be placed if they are not able or choose not to do so.[43] Though overcoming the effects of structural violence through community involvement sounds like a wonderful goal, it slights the realities of individuals' lives.

This might explain why Oak Park and Chatham exhibited different abilities to bounce back from the 2008 recession. Though both communities display high levels of social cohesion and collective efficacy, Oak Park is home to economically and socially privileged residents, many of whom are white. Chatham's collective efficacy may be strong compared to that of its surrounding neighborhoods, but this can do only so much to propel the community upward from a triple threat of economic decline, racism, and lack of health care access.

Overall, the idea of collective efficacy and community development is easy to romanticize—a close-knit, caring neighborhood sounds like a wonderful idea. However, it is necessary to consider such concepts with caution. The fact that collective efficacy and social cohesion may be associated with improved health outcomes does not mean they alone can be held out a solution to the current dismal state of concentrated poverty and health inequity in the United States.

Geography Matters

What, then, can be done? Is one solution simply to move as many people as possible, as Windora's sister Cora did, from high-stress communities of concentrated disadvantage to communities of concentrated advantage? In lower-stress and lower-poverty environments, does health really improve? While it is difficult to run controlled trials on neighborhood effects on health, there is some evidence that moving from a neighborhood of concentrated poverty to a better neighborhood does have lasting health benefits.

The Moving to Opportunity (MTO) experiment tested this hypothesis.[44] This was an outgrowth of the *Gautreaux* case, the first successful housing-discrimination lawsuit in US history. This case demonstrated that the Chicago Housing Authority and the US Department of Housing and Urban Development (HUD) violated the civil rights of poor black public-housing residents from 1950 to 1964 in their placement of high-rise public housing units in black inner-city neighborhoods.[45] Of the 10,300 HUD-constructed public housing units in Chicago, only 63 were built outside poor, racially segregated areas. This pattern of racially segregated public housing projects was the norm across the

United States. As a remedy, HUD designed and developed the MTO project to test the impact of neighborhood mobility on employment, income, education, and well-being.[46]

Families with children living in Baltimore, Boston, Chicago, Los Angeles, and New York in selected public housing developments and census tracts—with at least 40 percent of residents with incomes below the poverty threshold in 1990—were eligible to participate in a local housing-authority lottery for rent-subsidy vouchers. Nearly 4,500 participating families were randomly assigned to one of three groups. The first group was offered vouchers for housing in a census tract with a low poverty rate, along with housing counseling services. In the second group, families also received vouchers but with no restrictions on where they could reside. Families in the third, control group were offered no vouchers.[47]

The MTO experiment study had many limitations. In the first group, only about half used the vouchers. In the second group, a little under two-thirds used them. Furthermore, while those in the first group were encouraged to move to low-poverty middle-class neighborhoods, after only one year many returned to high-poverty neighborhoods similar to the ones they left. Nevertheless, the census-tract poverty rate for the first group was 17.1 percentage points lower than that for the control group, for which the poverty rate was 50.0 percent.[48]

The health outcomes associated with moving out of a high-poverty neighborhood were notable. Overall, families who received vouchers experienced better health benefits than those in the control group— particularly lower obesity and better-controlled diabetes.[49] Additionally, they were more likely to self-report better well-being.[50] In some localities, particularly in Yonkers, New York, the participants showed marked positive health effects of moving from high- to low-poverty neighborhoods.[51] Two years after single mothers and their sons moved to Yonkers, they reported better mental and physical health than did those who remained in high-poverty neighborhoods.[52] With more desirable housing conditions—better heating and air quality, less crowding, less exposure to violence, and fewer pest infestations—residents were less likely to experience stress, depression, or anxious behavior as well as other conditions, such as asthma, fatigue, or exposure to carcinogens.[53]

While MTO has its critics, it is clear ten to fifteen years later that those who received any type of housing voucher and moved away from concentrated poverty experienced significant health benefits.[54] People's material conditions can be improved, and that can mitigate their mental and physical health problems—a conclusion Cora would endorse.

Geography may matter in other ways as well. The poor in some cities—including New York City, San Francisco, and Los Angeles—live nearly as long as their better-off neighbors or at least have experienced rising life expectancies.[55] But in other parts of the country such as Gary (Indiana) and Detroit, adults with the lowest incomes die on average at the same age as people in much poorer nations, like Sudan and Ghana.[56] Poor people at the lowest 5 percent of the income scale in Gary will live five years less than those at the bottom 5 percent in New York City. Their life spans are getting shorter even compared to other poor Americans. We know that the social gradient of income inequality predicts mortality, but the idea that geography predicts life expectancy as well is a relatively recent concept. It makes sense that social cohesion and collective efficacy may vary region to region across America, just as they do from neighborhood to neighborhood in Chicago. Public health policies (a form of regional collective efficacy) that regulate food, smoking, and the environment are hypothesized to be at the root of this geographic variation. New York, Los Angeles, and San Francisco have more developed safety-net and public health systems, and this might account for the life-expectancy improvements seen there.

In these observations about communities, collective efficacy, and mortality variation, there is good news. Inequality and premature mortality are not inevitable. We have examples of communities like Oak Park and Chatham and regions like New York City and San Francisco that have mitigated the impact of structural violence on longevity by community action. These public policy changes that contribute to improved life expectancy for the poor in these regions could have been achieved only with the active engagement of community members and their political leaders fighting on behalf of their well-being.

COMMUNITY ACTIVISM AGAINST STRUCTURAL VIOLENCE

I have learned over the years that when one's mind is made up, this diminishes fear; knowing what must be done does away with fear.[1]

ROSA PARKS

Equity in health care cannot be achieved simply by the actions of legislatures, doctors, nurses, and health care organizations. As we saw in chapter 11, one measure of collective efficacy and social cohesion is an activated community ready to organize and act on its own behalf. Such a community can be a powerful tool for health improvement. Communities that are interested in the health of their members and demonstrate this through community participation may be healthier communities in the long run.[2] A sense of purpose, so critical to personal health, can also be important to improve community health.

In the absence of national or statewide policies to address health injustice, health inequity conflicts become local. The battlegrounds in these conflicts are often hospitals, clinics, insurance companies, and government agencies. Not surprisingly, Chicago has been ground zero for a number of churning health controversies. The transplant activism discussed in chapter 8 is one example.[3] Environmental activists, stirred by high pediatric asthma mortality in the area, forced the mothballing of coal-fired toxin-spewing power plants in Chicago.[4] The shuttering of public mental health clinics was accompanied by public outrage, demonstrations, and arrests.[5]

While health care institutions naturally try to avoid public confrontations about policies and practices, at times these skirmishes are unavoidable. Public actions directed against health institutions can be disruptive, but at the same time they foster opportunities for substantive structural improvements. Partnerships between communities and institutions are critical to overcome the structural and social conditions that precipitate premature mortality. While contentious conflicts between disadvantaged communities and powerful institutions can be painful, common cause, when achieved, can improve health.

In this chapter, against a backdrop of neglected and violence-torn neighborhoods, I spotlight a battle between a local black youth group demanding a Level 1 trauma center and the University of Chicago, a bastion of academic prowess.[6] The fight for a trauma center was linked to citywide activism over the decline of health and the implosion of poor neighborhoods in the wake of the Great Recession. An epidemic of gun violence in Chicago and a rash of highly publicized police-brutality cases fueled feelings of disenfranchisement among the youth. Two separate realities fanned the conflict: the business priorities of a successful, internationally renowned university medical center and the moral demands of members of a violence-stricken, poverty-afflicted neighboring black community. The battle zone was Chicago's South Side, but the conflict eventually breached the portals of the White House.[7]

Community Activists Target Health Care

The underlying neighborhood conditions on the South and West Sides of Chicago that have contributed to disease burden and premature mortality have also spawned a new generation of community activists. The years from 2010 through 2015 saw a flurry of this community activism around the issues of health care delivery, mental health, school closings, and public safety.[8] Spawned by an epidemic of gun violence and fueled by long-standing mistrust between the communities and institutions like the police, city hall, and health care infrastructure, the activism caught the city by surprise.

But these outbursts were more than a series of disconnected events.

Rather, they reflected the growing frustration of people living in long-neglected neighborhoods. Simmering grievances and injustices needed airing. The residents of these inner-city areas had watched their neighborhoods deteriorate since the middle part of the twentieth century. Despite fair housing laws, blacks are still preferentially steered by realtors to black neighborhoods with overpriced housing and are forced to pay what has been called a "race tax": the increased cost of goods and services from food to insurance to gasoline.[9]

Underserved by banks, these neighborhoods had been targeted by the harsh terms and high interest rates of predatory subprime lenders in the latter part of the twentieth century. Like unscrupulous ghetto contract lenders of the 1950s, subprime lenders strong-armed people into taking on risky debt. These neighborhoods were then pummeled by the mortgage loan crisis that caused the Great Recession in 2008. Foreclosures ravaged poor African American and Latino neighborhoods in particular.[10] In sixteen poor black Chicago neighborhoods, 10 percent of the homes were in foreclosure.[11] Boarded-up houses blighted residential neighborhoods, inviting drug dealing and vandalism. The devastation crippled even middle-class neighborhoods. The Bronzeville neighborhood recovered more slowly than other middle-class black neighborhoods in the nation, such as Harlem.[12] Black families, stripped of jobs, homes, cars, retirement accounts, and savings, saw wealth gains of a lifetime wiped out.[13] By 2011 black median household net worth had nosedived to $7,113.[14] (By comparison, the average white household's wealth was $111,146.)[15] Half the collective wealth of African American families was obliterated during the Great Recession.[16] It was an economic calamity of stupendous proportions and perhaps the largest drain on black American wealth ever recorded.[17] But this wealth death spiral failed to gain the attention of a nation as did police shootings of black men in many of the same affected neighborhoods in 2014 and 2015.[18]

#BlackLivesMatter and Community Health Activism

On Black Friday 2015, thousands of #BlackLivesMatter demonstrators disrupted Christmas shopping on Michigan Avenue in response to a

Autopsy Report: LaQuan McDonald

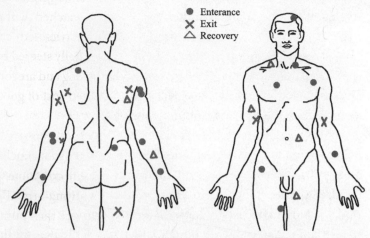

LaQuan McDonald was a mentally ill young black man who was shot sixteen times by the Chicago Police in October 2014. After the homicide was covered up for a time, an investigation of the police department found a pattern of discriminatory practices. Source: Office of the Medical Examiner, County of Cook.

Chicago city hall cover-up of the police murder of teenager Laquan McDonald.[19] McDonald's death was one of many well-publicized police shootings of young black men across the United States that spawned the #BlackLivesMatter movement in 2014.[20] McDonald, a troubled seventeen-year-old, was shot sixteen times by a police officer. A police conspiracy to cover up the murder ensued and eventually reached Mayor Rahm Emanuel at city hall. Fourteen months after the murder, an investigative reporter forced the city to release the video of it. It shocked the city and nation.[21] Police homicide and brutality were not new phenomena. Police have enforced structural violence and the criminalization of black life across America for generations. What was new was video evidence of police brutality and the way it could now travel via viral social media. The invisible was now visible.

The crowd of demonstrators included members of a South Side community organization named STOP, Southside Together Organizing for Power, and its youth organization, Fearless Leading by the Youth.[22] STOP and FLY led fights for housing equity and access to health care. The connection between the national movement and the local issues could not be any clearer to them. After all, the #BlackLives movement was not just about racist police violence. It was about long-standing structural violence and inequity.

Race, Place, and Policing

The tension between Chicago's black communities and the police had long simmered. For years Commander John Burge and his squad of detectives had tortured black prisoners into confessions in a South Side police station, yet the city defended him and other abusers in the face of lawsuits.[23] Between 2007 and 2012, Chicago police shot over four hundred people.[24] There were seventy police fatalities during that period, the most in the nation. Between 2004 and 2014, the cash-strapped city dished out $662 million in police brutality settlements.[25] Imagine how those funds might have helped failing schools or the health-care safety net. In April 2016, an independent investigative report declared the Chicago Police Department to be systematically racist, an assertion that was no surprise to residents.[26] Three-quarters of the police shootings and 72 percent of the use of tasers have been directed at black people.[27]

"The video that depicted the death of Laquan McDonald motivated a movement, and it was a tipping point, but really again the conversation about the narrative of the intersection of race and policing goes back decades," said Lori Lightfoot, chair of the Police Accountability Taskforce, which released the report.[28]

Meanwhile, an epidemic of gun violence targeting teenagers and young adults plagued the same Chicago neighborhoods affected by racist policing practices. What the neighborhoods needed was safety. The violence epidemic in these high-poverty neighborhoods was a five-alarm public health emergency. While some teen violence prevention programs, such as Cure Violence, have reduced repeat gun violence by 40 to 71 percent in some neighborhoods, the scope of the crisis is far greater than these programs can handle.[29] The root of the violence epidemic is structural violence: the lack of jobs, limited educational opportunities, the loss of wealth, and the loss of hope and purpose in these neighborhoods.

We can best understand the fight for a South Side trauma center in the context of this precipitous neighborhood decline, on top of generations of neighborhood neglect. In 2012 the city's decision to shutter six of twelve long-standing mental health clinics—four of them on the South Side—spawned wide protests and many arrests. County sheriff Tom Dart, who has described his jail as the state's "largest mental health provider," opposed the closings. "This is not higher math," Dart said. "If you reduce programs and remove funding, it isn't as if fairy dust will be spread throughout the clouds and these people's mental health issues will go away. They will still have them, and it's a question of where they will go from there. The majority are coming to the criminal justice system."[30]

STOP and other groups protested the closings, which the city claimed would save $3 million yearly.[31] The need for mental health services in the community was enormous—and growing even as the funding evaporated. This tension between money and need would fuel the trauma debate.

From the perspective of neighborhood leaders, the five-year battle for a Level 1 trauma center was not a one-issue battle. They had witnessed the besieging of their neighborhoods by losses of wealth and life, clinic and school closures, and the dimming of their children's prospects. The best efforts of the University of Chicago Hospitals to provide community health to the South Side was no match for the expectations of young black people who had to contend with the ravages of day-to-day violence in their communities.

Damian Turner Is Shot

A random shooting in 2010 triggered the demand for a South Side trauma center. Fifty-eight Chicagoans were shot that August, two fewer than the number of Americans killed in Iraq that entire year.[32] Damian Turner was one of them. A stray bullet pierced his 18-year-old chest in a drive-by shooting just four blocks from the University of Chicago Hospital. Wounded and bleeding, he staggered to his sister's nearby apartment and collapsed on her doorstep. She raced to the phone and called 911. The paramedics arrived and transported Damian to Northwestern Memorial Hospital, the closest trauma center, ten miles away. He was pronounced dead an hour after arrival. His family and friends were left wondering whether his life could have been saved had he been taken just a few blocks, to the University of Chicago.[33]

"Nobody on this earth deserves to die if they have a chance to live," Turner's mother, Sheila Rush, said to a reporter from *The Nation*. "My son did not even have a chance, because he was fighting for his life on the way in that ambulance on that long ride to the hospital."[34]

The University of Chicago had closed down its adult trauma unit twenty-five years prior, when it was hemorrhaging $2 million a year.[35] The university maintained a pediatric trauma center but admitted teenage trauma victims only up to the age of 15. Located in the middle-class Hyde Park neighborhood, the hospital is flanked by black neighborhoods where gun violence is rampant. Mistrust between the university and the black South Side had festered for seventy-five years because the community interpreted the university's urban development practices as a tool to blunt black intrusion into Hyde Park. In the 1930s, a Metropolitan Chicago Housing and Planning Council (MHPC) composed of white real estate and banking interests was formed to address "urban blight" just as blacks were flowing into the city's neighborhoods. The council steered into law the Illinois Blighted Areas Redevelopment Act, which pioneered the concept of "urban renewal." The law created and empowered a Land Clearance Commission to use eminent domain to acquire land in "blighted" areas, demolish the existing buildings, then sell the land at steep discounts to private investors. *Urban blight* became a code phrase to justify the dismantling of black neighborhoods that encroached on white neighborhoods and business districts. Black neighborhoods were thus disproportionally targeted for redevelopment. The city council doubled down on this scheme by passing legislation to keep public housing that was open to black people from being located in white neighborhoods. These laws inspired federal urban-renewal legislation that replicated the Chicago plan across the United States, but also provided funding for black neighborhood destruction. Black people displaced by urban renewal and blocked from white wards were forced to take refuge in dense, overcrowded black neighborhoods. One neighborhood that attracted new black apartment dwellers and homeowners in the 1940s was Hyde Park.[36]

In the late 1940s, University of Chicago officials feared that they might lose their student base if the neighborhood became black. Working with the MHPC, they engineered a piece of state (and eventually federal) housing legislation that allowed neighborhoods that were not yet "blighted" to be razed by targeting what were euphemistically called "pockets of decay"—in other words, black neighborhoods. By 1958 the "conservation" of the Hyde Park neighborhood had destroyed perfectly fine housing in the black southwest side of the neighborhood. The urban renewal plan called for the destruction of 20 percent of Hyde Park's housing and the removal of 20,000 black residents without any relocation plans. Over the next fifty years university efforts to clear "blight" in the neighborhoods surrounding Hyde Park fanned the tension between neighborhood residents and the university.[37]

While the University of Chicago Hospital officials thought they were making a simple business decision about whether to offer trauma services, some black neighbors interpreted the decision through the historical prism of mistrust and perceived racial discrimination by the university. In 2009 some claimed that the university was trying to deflect routine care of the local community to other institutions by limiting emergency room care, a move that was widely condemned.[38] The university hospital is the only major hospital on the South Side. It boasts a deep bench of medical and surgical specialists. The other hospitals are essentially small safety-net institutions with limited services and shaky finances. If you are sick on the South Side, the University of Chicago Hospital is the best place to go.

When Damian Turner died, his murder awakened long-dormant grievances held by some black South Siders against the university. Turner was a popular community youth leader and a cofounder of FLY, an organization composed of high school and college-age students. At the time of his murder, the group had been working to improve the living conditions of kids detained in the city's Youth Detention Facility. When FLY leaders assembled to mourn Damian's death, they shared memories of other friends who had perished from gunshots. In these discussions they identified the lack of South Side trauma care as a public health issue. They believed that if the University of Chicago had a trauma center, Damian would not have died. So FLY publicly asked the university to open a trauma center.[39] On what would have been Damian's nineteenth birthday, FLY activists held a demonstration in front of the university hospital to reiterate their demand and request a meeting with the university leadership. Five years passed before the medical center leader agreed to meet. Yet FLY leaders, undaunted by the challenge ahead and determined to honor the memory of their fallen leader, chanted at every rally and meeting, "I believe that we will win!"

For its part, the university maintained that Chicago had no need for another trauma center and to build one would be cost-prohibitive. Both positions were accurate. There was plenty of trauma capacity at the regional trauma centers. As *The Nation* later described the situation:

> Chicago's four trauma centers are located on the city's west and north sides. The Southside of Chicago where most of the gunshots victims were being injured had no adult trauma center. Dr. Gary Merlotti, the chief of trauma at Sinai Health System on the Westside, noted that the city suffered from neither an insufficient quantity nor quality of trauma centers. "I don't think we have an inadequate number," Merlotti says. "We have a geographic maldistribution."[40]

The finances of trauma care are dismal. Most trauma centers lose money, as many patients are uninsured. For FLY's new leader Darius Lightfoot, the issue was not revenue but the value of black lives. "Show us that you really care. Show us that you really value a black life," he said.[41]

FLY understood the issue as a crisis of morality and health justice, as well as a test of the university's commitment to the black South Side. The medical center leaders saw it as a question of resource utilization. But it was difficult to frame the debate as simply a resource question in light of the national #BlackLives movement and the depth of racial inequities in Chicago. FLY's demands extended beyond trauma care. FLY sought a broader program to address the health issue of greatest concern to the community: violence.

Alex Goldenberg, executive director of STOP (FLY's parent organization), explained the connection:

> We definitely see gun violence cutting across a number of other issues. The fight for trauma care allows you to talk about these issues. We're not asking just for the care but we are really fighting to change the whole continuum of issues that violence is resulting in. At one end of the spectrum you have the trauma center, which is leading for the care for the injury. But you also have the violence interrupter that's there with the friends, family, relatives and the person who is injured. Then there are the services to follow up with the family and friends. Then you have all the other needed things like jobs and after school programs that support prevention. The coalition we are building is fighting for all of those things.[42]

The activists organized students, religious leaders, not-for-profits, physicians, and other health professionals under an umbrella Trauma Care Coalition.

Change Starts to Come

Over five years, three independent events contributed to the medical center's reversal of its position. The first was the 2013 grand opening of its $700 million high-tech, gleaming hospital bed tower, the Center for Care and Discovery, in 2013. The tower's state-of-the-art magnificence contrasts with the poverty of surrounding neighborhoods. For community members who feel locked out, it symbolizes the wealth gaps and structural inequities that they experience every day. After the new hospital opened, the medical center found it difficult to use cost as an argument against building a trauma center. "The optics were kind of absurd," said Alex Goldenberg.[43]

FLY disrupted the building's opening by signing up for a public tour and then holding a sit-in in the lobby. Batons swinging, University of Chicago police cleared the demonstrators and arrested four people. Shortly afterward the medical center dean announced that the hospital would study a regional strategy for a trauma center—the first glimpse that a victory might be possible. Many demonstrations and prayer sessions followed, with police dragging protestors from a construction site in 2014 and clearing praying protestors from the hospital's lobby at other times. In June 2015, nine protestors were arrested after barricading themselves in a university building.[44]

An influential study by Northwestern trauma surgeon Marie Crandall, in the June 2013 journal of the American Public Health Association, helped FLY's cause, calling Chicago's South Side a trauma care desert.[45] Crandall's study illuminated the extent to which the maldistribution of trauma care posed a deadly threat to a subset of patients. Studying gunshot wounds in Chicago, she found higher mortality among people who traveled more than five miles for trauma care than among those who traveled fewer than five miles—particularly patients with wounds like those of Damian Turner.[46] *The Nation* estimated that almost a fifth of Chicago residents live five or more miles away from a trauma center, most of them on the black South Side. More than a third of the city's homicides and shootings between 2001 to 2013 have unfolded more than five miles away from a trauma center.[47] Crandall's study provided evidence that sanctioned FLY's and Turner's family's suspicions that delay and distance might contribute to death. Studies beyond Chicago have not proved that distance factors in trauma mortality. But given that Crandall's study was specifically based on Chicago's data, it was hard to argue with her conclusions.

The third factor that may have tipped the scales was the US president himself. In 2014 the University of Chicago and the City of Chicago lobbied for the Obama Presidential Library to be located near campus. Trauma-center protestors seized the opportunity, organizing events and chanting "No trauma, no Bama." Soon influential community leaders conditioned their support for the Obama Library on the building of a trauma center.[48] The university's pursuit of the Obama Library may have forced it to concede on the trauma center.

The University of Chicago Medical Center faced internal pressure about trauma care as well. Many medical students, medical faculty, nurses, and staff supported the Trauma Coalition's demand and urged the administration to concede. The moral suasion of the university community was at the very least a factor in the eventual decision.

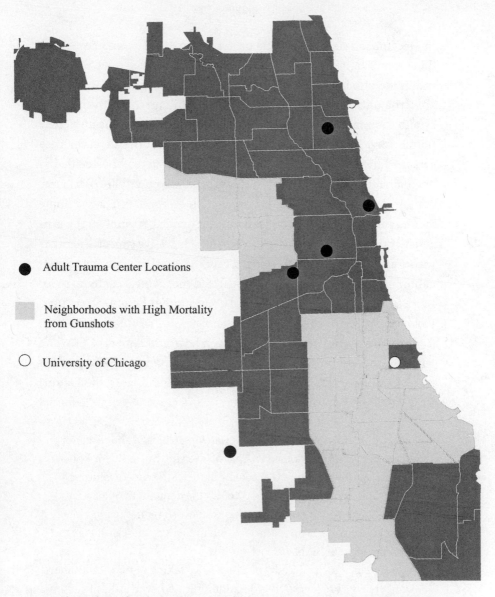

Adult Trauma Center Locations

Neighborhoods with High Mortality
from Gunshots

University of Chicago

On Chicago's South Side there are no adult trauma centers within the neighborhoods hardest hit by gunshot mortality. Gunshot victims have been forced to travel out of the neighborhoods, bypassing the University of Chicago Hospital, which treats trauma only up to the age of 15. Community activists, led by high school students, convinced the university to open an adult trauma center after years of demonstrations that garnered national attention. Source: *Crain's Chicago Business*, 2010.

Victory for the South Side

In December 2014, the medical center leaders began stutter-stepping their way to a decision. They announced that the age for pediatric trauma treatment would be raised from 15 to 17. Then in September 2015, the university announced that it would partner with the Sinai Health System to build a trauma center five miles west of the university hospital on a Sinai hospital property. In December 2015, however, they scrapped the deal with Sinai and announced that they had decided to open an adult trauma center on their own campus as part of a larger commitment to expand health care services on the South Side.[49] Some viewed the expansion announcement as a cynical attempt by the university to improve its finances by providing lucrative cancer and other medical care in addition to trauma care.[50] But others saw it as a welcome and genuine about-face that will lead the medical center to focus more fully on the complex needs of communities beset by structural violence.

The voice of the community had been heard. Members of FLY and STOP were cautiously optimistic that a trauma center would be built but will remain wary until it opens.[51] On December 15, 2015, the Trauma Care Coalition released a statement:

> In this moment, the whole world is watching Chicago and its history and practice of institutional racism. The decision by President Robert Zimmer and Dean Kenneth Polonsky of the University of Chicago to listen to the community and concede to the demand to open a Level I Adult Trauma Center and save black lives shows that young black people can absolutely impact policy and influence political change for the betterment of the black community.
>
> We applaud the University of Chicago for taking responsibility as a member of the broader south side community. A Level I Adult Trauma Center at the University of Chicago will provide the best possible outcome for addressing the current lack of south side trauma care. It also signals a significant shift in the University's approach to responding to the needs of its predominantly Black South Side neighbors....
>
> This is a movement moment. We are winning and need to dream

bigger and demand more to create a society where healthcare is a human right and all human rights are respected. We are calling on everyone who has struggled with us and all oppressed people to dream bigger. Let's do more, it's working, we can get the things that we want. The "I believe that we will win" chant is not just a chant, it is real.[52]

OBSERVE, JUDGE, ACT

Ultimately a great nation is a compassionate nation. America has not met its obligations and its responsibilities to the poor. One day we will have to stand before the God of history and we will talk in terms of things we've done. Yes, we will be able to say we built gargantuan bridges to span the seas, we built gigantic buildings to kiss the skies.... It seems that I can hear the God of history saying, "That was not enough! But I was hungry, and ye fed me not. I was naked, and ye clothed me not. I was devoid of a decent sanitary house to live in, and ye provided no shelter for me...." This is America's opportunity to help bridge the gulf between the haves and the have-nots. The question is whether America will do it.[1]

MARTIN LUTHER KING JR.

Observe, Judge, Act

It would not suffice for me to diagnose inequality as a cause of America's premature mortality and death gaps without offering a prescription for cure, any more than it would suffice for a firefighter to witness a three-alarm blaze without grabbing a hose. For my prescription I turn to the insights of Dr. Paul Farmer, the humanitarian physician whose work in Haiti, Rwanda, Peru, and Russia with his human rights group, Partners in Health, has been at the forefront of treating the maladies of the poor caused by structural violence. In his book *Pathologies of Power*, Farmer wrote about three precepts that have guided his health justice work around the world: observe, judge, and act.[2] These precepts are critical to grasp to solve the problem of inequality as a cause of premature American death. Observe what is happening. Analyze it. Judge the reasons why people are dying prematurely. Then act. These three precepts were first introduced in 1930 by the Belgian cardinal Joseph Cardijin, then promoted by Pope John XXIII in his encyclical letter *Mater et Magistra* in 1961.[3] They were widely adopted in Latin America as a thread of liberation theology and in Chicago by antiracist priests fighting redlining, blockbusting, and other acts of structural violence.[4] They are meant as a guide to follow to translate social justice principles into action.

Observe

Medicine has a clear obligation to work on behalf of the poor but often falls short in the United States—indeed, across the world. With its focus on profit margins, the American health care system has directed the tools of biomedical technology to preferentially benefit the rich and middle class at the expense of the health needs of the poor. Because health care is a commodity and not considered a human right in the United States, the poor inevitably suffer.

We have developed a polite vernacular that allows us to avoid the scandalous conditions of health inequality in our midst. Using euphemisms like "poor payer-mix" allows health system administrators to avoid delivering direct service to poor and minority neighborhoods. We tend to build clinics and high-technology centers in wealthier (and often white) neighborhoods. We avoid some of the Medicaid insurance plans that cover the poor, because they don't pay us well. We limit the uninsured access to our clinics and technology. Our doctors and administrators are from largely white and privileged neighborhoods and often have little insight into the day-to-day lives of their poorest patients. While some of our institutions and many physicians do their best to serve the sick and poor, their service falls short of the need. We have too long tolerated rich-poor, white-minority inequities in treatments and health care outcomes. We have pretended that separate health care for the poor is equal to the care for the middle class and the rich. It is not.

Physicians are the "natural attorneys" for the poor, uniquely po-sitioned to advocate on their behalf. Yet too often we have remained silent as our hospitals and insurance companies have pursued material gain over solving the health needs of patients in our most troubled communities. Most of us are uncomfortable acknowledging the bru-tal truth of life and death in America—that much suffering and early death stem from social and economic conditions and are preventable. Most of us, even if we acknowledge the unnecessary deaths, do not feel comfortable speaking up. It is uniquely the province of medicine to observe and ameliorate the conditions affecting populations suffering in ill health and poverty. One could argue that the disproportionate burden of disease and premature mortality inflicted on the poor obliges medicine to preferentially serve, care, and treat our most marginalized populations. To observe the state of health and low life expectancy in the poor requires that medicine not just heal the individual. It must address the social and economic conditions that elicit and aggravate illness. Take for instance, the visit of Mr. M to my office.

A Suicide Attempt

Mr. M is a 62-year-old black man. He looks ten years older, with cropped gray hair and a heavily wrinkled face with deep-set walnut-colored eyes and silver stubble on his cheeks and chin. He's been my patient for a few years and suffers from diabetes, cirrhosis of the liver, emphysema, hypertension, and arthritis. An ex-offender, he is living a precarious hand-to-mouth existence in the inner city. Usually we discuss his diabetes or his chronic pain. But today he told me that he had tried to kill himself. I stopped typing into the electronic chart, slid back on my rolling stool, and turned to face him.

As he told his story, the pained look on his face contrasted with the bright gleam of my examination room with its wall rack of trendy magazines and an examination table centered on an antiseptic white tile floor. My current office sits within one city block of the cubicle where I saw my first outpatient in the summer of 1978. In these almost four decades of practicing primary care in this one Chicago neighbor-hood, I have observed over and over again the trauma that a lifetime of structural violence inflicts on the human body and soul. Today was no exception.

Mr. M had been acting erratically during the last month, and Megan, the nurse practitioner, thought that he might be using drugs.

"What happened to you?" I ask. "We were worried that something was wrong." I run through a standardized checklist of questions to assess whether Mr. M was depressed. When I ask him if he has thoughts of suicide, he nods.

"I thought I needed to kill myself," he says. "'Forget this. I am outta here.'" He described his physical pain and his shortness of breath. "Stuff is coming to me from everywhere. I can't move like I used to. I am short of breath and in pain all the time. I need to leave here."

Mr. M is also homeless. He moves from shelter to shelter, from street to street, day in and day out. He was evicted from his last apartment and owes $1,400 in back rent. There is not a stable housing option on his horizon anytime soon, so he wanders with his possessions from place to place.

"So I went to a guy I knew who sold heroin, and I snorted some because I wanted to end it. Everything was too much for me. The way I was living. I'm sick, myself. Then I watched my mom have a heart attack. My brother is an alcoholic and all he wants to do is fight all the time. I did not want to live no more. Someone found me and called the ambulance. I was taken to Swedish [a Chicago hospital]. I came back to my senses after that."

"Why did you want to kill yourself?" I ask.

"I have my own stress," he says. "Then I have the stress in my family, trying to hold them together. Then there is the stress in the streets, trying to maneuver around to avoid this person or that street. The stress is so much sometimes that it makes me feel like my head is going to bust. It is the fear that I feel all the time. Sometimes I feel like giving up. I just want to lay down and die."

Doctors can be overwhelmed by the sheer magnitude of the distress and disease burdens that target the poor. Those of us who provide health care for the poor often encounter patients like Mr. M, living in the midst of despair. All of us have witnessed the crippling impact of grinding poverty on our patients. It's not just the premature mortality.

It's the burden of living with disease and distress on a day-to-day basis. There is not a pill for Mr. M's misery. However, safe and affordable housing might have prevented his suicide attempt. All I had to offer was a willing ear to listen, a social work referral, and an offer to see him again in a couple of weeks.

I have been at this for a long time. It does not get easier. When one takes the time to peel back the doctor-patient relationship, a world is revealed that would be quite shocking to the average middle-class American. Yet we are all a bankruptcy, a job loss, a catastrophic illness away from a life of misery ourselves. I wish I could report that the lives of the poor have materially improved in my decades as a doctor in Chicago. By many measures they are worse.

We recently analyzed the causes for hospitalizations in the West Side neighborhoods just beyond my hospital's portals. In most neighborhoods of concentrated advantage people go to the hospital to deliver babies or to get cardiac treatments and the like. But in the neighborhoods of high hardship, the top reason for hospitalization is mental illness. An epidemic of mental illness caused by the social and economic conditions in Chicago's inner-city neighborhoods. Mr. M is just the latest victim.

Judge

To judge requires we accurately assess the root cause of America's death gaps. I have named structural violence as a critical driver of health inequality.

Not behaviors.

Not biology.

Not culture.

Not bad luck.

But deliberate public and economic policies that have allowed inequality to flourish at the cost of life itself. That is not to reject individual responsibility and accountability for health outcomes. Or to deny that diseases have biological manifestations. But individual behaviors, biology, and culture are insufficient explanations for the neighborhood-to-neighborhood gaps in illness and life expectancy. And they deflect attention from the social, political, and economic fault lines that create survival gaps.

The Chicago Transit Authority Blue Line train has a stop just in front of my hospital. The life expectancy around the Blue Line stop in Chicago's Loop, just east of Rush University Hospital, is 85 years. Three stops down the Blue Line from Rush is Mr. M's neighborhood, where life expectancy plummets to less than 69. No measured assessment of the health conditions in America's neighborhoods could fail to connect the marginalized existence of so many and the economic structures and racial discrimination that have enriched many at the expense of the poor. Even if you don't agree that structural violence is the root cause of our neighborhood ills, there can be no doubt that something is dreadfully wrong. Neighborhood and life conditions have deteriorated to the point where they drive patients like Mr. M to madness and, worse, suicide.

And yet we are anesthetized by these neighborhood conditions. We have tolerated the wickedness of inequity as if it were a natural condition of a modern capitalist society. We avert our gaze so we do not have to endure the jarring emotional dissonance created by the juxtaposition of great wealth and mammoth poverty. Despite the evidence that structural violence inflicts terrible psychological stress on the poor, the City of Chicago's Health Department closed its mental health clinics a few years ago.[5] At the same time, Chicago's jails and emergency rooms overflow with the mentally ill. Under what measure of fairness and justice can this be justified?

Concentrated poverty and distress are mushrooming in the United States. For those on the short end of the wealth stick, the system is rigged. The negative impact of structural violence has skyrocketed as jobs, opportunities, and wealth have deserted more and more American neighborhoods in the twenty-first century. The United States now boasts more high-poverty neighborhoods in any time since the 1960s.[6] Since 2000, the number of people living in high-poverty ghettos and slums nearly doubled, from 7.2 million to 13.8 million, while poverty became more densely concentrated. More than one in four African

Americans and more than one in three Latinos now live in neighborhoods of extreme poverty. Contrast this to white America. One in thirteen white Americans lives in this concentrated poverty—nothing to celebrate, but disproportionate to the US black and Latino experience.[7]

Because white poverty is more dispersed than black and Latino poverty, the death gaps within the white community can be difficult to discern. While white America experiences better health overall than black America, some neighborhoods in white America are not inoculated against the impact of structural violence. An analysis by the *Washington Post* found that since 2000, American white women have been dying at higher rates expiring in their 30s, 40s, and 50s, an invisible crisis driven by the impact of postglobalization job loss on small-town America. In one of the hardest-hit groups—rural white women in their late 40s—the death rate has risen by 30 percent. As life has evolved in rural America, as jobs have been dispatched overseas, as poverty has swelled, more white men and women are dying prematurely.

A greater proportion of Americans lived in poverty in 2015—a staggering 45 million—than in the late 1960s. Children are the hardest hit, with almost half of them below five years old living in poverty.[8] Chicago is an epicenter for child distress, with the highest child poverty rate in the nation. While black and Latino men have been imprisoned at unprecedented rates, black women and their children have faced an epidemic of evictions because of poverty and racism.[9] The wealth gap between whites and minorities is the largest it has been since 1989.[10] The wealth gap for single women in America is even starker. Single black and Hispanic women have a median wealth of $100 and $120 respectively; the median for single white women is $41,500. Nearly half of all single black and Hispanic women have zero or negative wealth, meaning that their debts exceed their total assets. These statistics demonstrate graphic inequity, but we should not forget that the preponderance of poverty in the United States is among whites.[11]

We have performed enough analyses. There are no more observations or judgments to make. If we were studying the impact of structural violence on health and longevity in a randomized clinical trial, the experiment would have been halted long ago on ethical grounds. It is time to act. It is time for healing.

Act

We can act on behalf of the poor. We can choose to neither objectify nor dismiss their experiences. We can insist on and pursue their right for health and longevity. We can speak up against structural violence. We can demand political and policy solutions to mitigate or eliminate the structures that impart violence. We can advocate for a fair and equitable health-care system organized around the precept of health as a human right. We can expect our institutions to do more to serve the interests of America's high-poverty communities and their residents. We can expect our leaders and policy makers to hold all our institutions to greater accountability for the lives of the poor. Finally, we can act personally to preferentially serve the poor.

To speak against the forces of structural violence—racism; economic exploitation; mass incarceration; the lack of safety, good education, and decent-paying jobs—requires us to make the invisible visible. That means we have to acknowledge and address the distress in our high-hardship communities. We can seek to understand all the ways in which racial and anti-poor bias is explicitly and implicitly built into our institutions and then work to overcome these biases. To act against structural violence first requires us to expose the conditions that curtail life and hasten death in our midst.

During the 1960 presidential campaign, when John F. Kennedy visited coal-mining country in eastern Kentucky, he was so jarred by what he witnessed—"the hungry children, ... the old people who cannot pay their doctor's bills, the families forced to give up their farms"— that he pledged to take action.[12] At age eight, because of that visit, I confronted the faces of suffering and misery in the papers and on my living-room TV screen. The whole nation was moved to action, shocked by the abject poverty in the midst of American postwar prosperity. This revelation ultimately resulted in the War on Poverty, Medicare, Medicaid, Head Start, and other social programs that lifted the lives of millions of poor Americans and redistributed wealth back to the poor.[13]

Similarly, when #BlackLivesMatter activists descended on Ferguson, Missouri, and stood down law-enforcement officials in the summer of 2014, after the police murder of teenager Michael Brown, they made the invisible suffering within that community visible to the country and world.[14] To break the silence about the structural causes of poverty and discrimination is a necessary first step toward cure. It requires that we talk openly about structural violence as a root cause of health inequity and premature mortality in our nation. Political and policy action are required as well. A restructuring of American society is necessary to reverse the corrosive impact of structural violence on mortality. These structural reforms could take many forms, from tax and job policy to the ending of mass incarceration. From the perspective of health care reform, the adoption of a single-payer health care system is the only way to create equity in health care.[15] Single-payer health care will be vigorously opposed by the profit-driven private health insurers and by those who will insist it is too costly or not feasible. But those of us advocating for health and longevity for the poor must insist on an insurance system that is universal, free, and accessible to all. Such a system will also be a step toward a fairer distribution of wealth. But to achieve lasting equity will require more than single-payer health care. It will require a massive reinvestment of new jobs and educational opportunities into the United States' most distressed neighborhoods.

To challenge the structures that impart violence and perpetuate hardship is no easy task. After all, the forces of structural violence are mighty. They have deep historical roots. One cannot comprehend the misery experienced in inner-city black neighborhoods today without honoring the fact that that today's neighborhood conditions are historical products of a quarter of a millennium of brutal slavery, ninety years of Jim Crow peonage, decades of neighborhood segregation, discriminatory lending policies, poverty, and mass imprisonment.[16] One cannot note the suicides, the alcoholism, and the sub-Saharan life expectancy on Native American reservations like Pine Ridge without acknowledging the historical connection to the genocide of millions of Native Americans, followed by the exile of their remnants to desolate regions. One cannot note the soaring mortality rates from drug overdoses, suicide, and cirrhosis among poor white Americans without acknowledging the historical growth of vast income inequality and job loss in rural America caused by globalization and tax policies.[17]

The contours of health and life expectancy in the United States are shaped by these destructive historical forces and events. As a nation, we have never reconciled or collectively grieved the sins of our history, national origins, and economic success. There are restorations and reparations to be made.

There are more immediate ways medicine can act on behalf of the poor. We need to take these actions for a number of reasons. First, a prescription for social and economic injustice is not readily to hand. The reshaping of the balance of equity in American society is necessary but not likely to happen soon. Reversing the structural conditions that have caused poverty rates to skyrocket will require long-term political and policy changes. Finally, the structural and political conditions that culminate in premature death have never been motivated by a desire to oppress people for the sake of doing so. These have always been the ways that powerful interests have maintained their rule and accumulated wealth. This will not change overnight, and not without a fight. But medicine can act, even in the face of such massive social and structural obstacles, to ameliorate suffering and even cure. And as doctors and health professionals (and others) facing the maladies of the poor, we have an obligation and ability to heal now.

Most doctors across the world take the Hippocratic Oath as a public rite of passage into medicine. In the aftermath of World War II and the revelations of genocide and sadistic medical experimentation by Nazi physicians, the oath was revised (and thus is now sometimes called the Declaration of Geneva, Physicians Oath):

At the time of being admitted as a member of the medical profession:

I solemnly pledge to consecrate my life to the service of humanity;

I will give my teachers the respect and gratitude that is their due;

I will practice my profession with conscience and dignity;

The health of my patient will be my first consideration;

I will respect the secrets that are confided in me, even after the patient has died;

I will maintain by all the means in my power, the honor and noble traditions of the medical profession;

My colleagues will be my brothers and sisters;

I will not permit the considerations of age, disease or disability, creed, ethnic origin, gender, nationality, political affiliation, race, sexual orientation, social standing to intervene between my duty and my patient;

I will maintain the utmost respect for human life;

I will not use my medical knowledge to violate human rights and civil liberties, even under threat.

I make these promises solemnly, freely and upon my honor.[18]

It is a doctor's oath but one we can all aspire to live by. If we choose to live and practice by this oath, then we have a special responsibility to preferentially prevent and treat the diseases that afflict the poor. To offer our personal services as caregivers in service to the poor is a critical action even in the absence of major structural changes in society. For doctors and nurses who treat those experiencing great social hardship and illness, the simple act of healing is a way to create common cause and dispense hope. It is not a world-changing act but a powerful statement of alignment between the profession and the most oppressed in our midst.

While I focus on the responsibility of doctors under the Hippocratic Oath, this is not limited to doctors. We all, whether doctor, nurse, administrator, or layperson, have something we can do to mitigate suffering through personal advocacy. Unfortunately, there are many in the healing professions who are numbed to the suffering of the poor or grimace in uncomfortable silence when confronted with the harsh and seemingly unsolvable realities of life and death in America just beyond the four walls of their clinics. I am hopeful that one day the discussion of preventable premature deaths and their links to the social and economic conditions in American neighborhoods will be central to professional discourse and practice.

There is something else that preferential care on behalf of the poor allows. It has the possibility to create hope and a sense of common purpose between ourselves, our institutions, our patients, and their communities. We know that individuals who feel that their life has purpose live 15 percent longer than those without purpose.[19] I do not want to overstate the impact of acting preferentially on behalf of the poor in creating purpose and hope, but honoring the views of the community is critical to building trust and effect cure. Paul Farmer calls this *acting in pragmatic solidarity* with our patients and communities.

Farmer gives an example of pragmatic solidarity in describing the work of his organization, Partners in Health, in Haiti as he and his colleagues tried to understand why Haitian dirt farmers who had tuberculosis were resisting treatment. Some anthropologists thought these Haitians believed that tuberculosis was caused by spells cast by others and that their beliefs explained their refusal to take the medications. But Farmer found that the peasants themselves had a more logical explanation. When they took the tuberculosis medication, their condition improved, but they became very hungry. Since they had no food, they stopped taking the medications because the tuberculosis curbed their hunger. They explained their predicament regarding taking TB meds without food to Farmer in Creole, roughly translated this way: "It's like washing your hands and drying them in the dirt."[20] Once Partners in Health provided food with the medications, the patients were fully adherent. Farmer's point was that you did not have to change the Haitians' cultural beliefs to improve their health. But you did have to *listen to them and solve the problem in a manner consistent with their needs.*

There were many times when Windora Bradley's diabetes and blood pressure were out of control because she cut back on her medications. I discovered that she could not afford her medication copays and also pay to feed her children. At times, in pragmatic solidarity, I arranged to get her bill paid so she could get back on track. If medicine can act in solidarity with the poor by understanding and treating their social as well as medical needs, suffering can be mitigated; diseases cured, lives extended. Sometimes, though, there is no treatment to offer, and listening itself is the only act of solidarity available.

In the summer of 2012, three pre-med students and I visited a church in the Mexican American La Villita neighborhood, about a mile and a half from Rush. The congregants were all uninsured, undocumented immigrants in need of organ transplants. One after another they and their families pleaded their cases to me. Each story was more poignant than the one before. Marco was 19 and had developed renal failure at 17. He was tethered to dialysis three times a week. His life, his education, was on hold. His mother was with him and described through tears their family's anguish over Marco's illness. Blanca was 21 with a similar history. Gustavo was 38 on dialysis, and María was 54 with liver cirrhosis.

I spent two hours with the students at the church, witnessing the testimonies and taking notes. I had no transplants to offer. I came empty-handed even though there were three transplant centers within a few miles of the church. But as a doctor, I could listen.

In the car driving back to the hospital, I asked the students to debrief their observations of the church visit with me. One of them broke into sobs. "It's so unfair!" she cried.

And yes, it was so unfair. To witness the brutality of inequality can reduce one to tears. It is why medicine often opts to ignore the harsh reality of premature illness and death in high-poverty neighborhoods. It is difficult to witness misery without suffering oneself, especially when the solutions to health inequity are available but denied simply because of money. But sometimes the act of listening provides a little dose of hope to those in need.

Two weeks after our visit to La Villita, the congregants, demanding transplant access, held a rally at the University of Illinois Hospital.[21] My three students showed up to join the action. When the congregants recognized the students, they enveloped them with hugs and tears. The students' presence was an act of solidarity that validated the demonstrators' struggle. The students' witness was an affirmation that these undocumented patients and their hope for cure were not invisible.

Hope and purpose can be transmitted like a vaccination, a booster against despair. Hope does not cure disease, but it is palliative.

Three years later, many of these patients we encountered that afternoon at the church have received transplants. Family members or strangers donated organs for a number of them. Some have become my patients at my institution. Marco received a kidney donated by his brother and is now in college. His mother and brother are now my patients. Gustavo and another undocumented patient, María, each received a kidney transplant the same day at my hospital. The family of a dying patient in Houston saw a story about these undocumented transplant patients and directly donated both kidneys when the patient passed. The three students, now all in medical school, will carry the lesson of that visit in the church forward in their medical careers.

But there is even more that we must do to act on behalf of the poor. It is our job to set the moral standards high for ourselves and our institutions. Too often our avoidance and passivity fails the poor. We do not speak up on their behalf. We do not allow the stories of our patients' privation and injustice to be amplified through our voices. If one solution to health inequality is a system of true universal health care as a fundamental human right, it starts when we make demands on our own practices and institutions to do more to serve the poor and uninsured. To do this is not that difficult. But it does require that we ask ourselves and institutional leaders at every critical medical center decision, How is this decision relevant to the suffering of the poor and to the relief of that suffering? If we can align our institutional practices to answer this question, we will make progress in eliminating neighborhood life-expectancy gaps.

It is critical that doctors see their responsibility to be advocates for the human rights of their patients wherever they work. These conversations are necessary and uplifting for health care organizations, most of which were founded on moral grounds to serve those in need. But these organizations can lose their moorings in the murky world of health care finances and insurance politics. There is a business imperative to health care delivery, but hospitals that act as holding companies and profit centers while denying the poor the human right to health care have lost their way. Demands by doctors, health care workers, and the public on behalf of the poor can help redirect such organizations back to their healing missions to the benefit of all. Medicine is human rights work. It is what we took an oath to uphold. But only if we all act.

As physicians, health care workers, or just everyday people interested in justice and fairness, we have an obligation to speak up politically to improve access to health care for all. At the time of this writing, there are nineteen states into which the Affordable Care Act has not expanded. Because of this, the black uninsured rate is twice what would be otherwise.[22] Because half of black America lives in nonexpansion states, 1.4 million blacks—23 percent of the nation's black uninsured population—have been prevented from getting insurance.[23] Meanthile, the health care marketplaces are failing to reduce out-of-pocket costs for the middle class across the country. The system is a flawed, crazy mess. But we need to fight on our patients' behalf for full implementation of the Affordable Care Act while we campaign for a universal single-payer solution to replace it.

Anchor Missions for Community Health

Finally, hospitals and health systems can serve the poor more fully. Our institutions can preferentially serve the poor by adopting a mission to treat all patients regardless of ability to pay. They can expand access for the poor by accepting the insurance plans used by the poor. They can measure and eliminate health care disparities within their health facilities and offices. There is a fledgling recognition by health care systems across the United States that their traditional approach to health care delivery will not reduce the health gaps in our communities of concentrated poverty. Business as usual will not reverse the epidemic of ill health and high mortality in our neighborhoods. A few systems have recognized that they will have to tackle the structural and social determinants of health. This is a new concept, and one with great implications.[24]

Because traditional industry and wealth have abandoned neighborhoods in urban and rural regions alike, hospitals are often among the largest employers in their communities. Health systems are a form of sticky capital, with billions of dollars flowing in and out of their communities each year, rather than to a distant corporate headquarters. In each of the twenty largest cities in America, hospitals and universities are among the top ten employers. Hospitals are also proximate to neighborhoods of concentrated poverty and hardship. America's inner cities are home to 350 hospitals and about one in fifteen of the nation's largest hospitals.[25] What if the mission of our nation's health systems were shifted to generate economic and health returns aimed to revitalize neighborhoods? Hospitals and health systems can use their heft as employers and as purchasers to bring jobs and other resources to the high-mortality, high-poverty neighborhoods in their environs. To do this, they need to see themselves as anchors responsible for the overall well-being of people in those neighborhoods. This goes beyond traditional hospital-based community-service programs and represents a conscious application of resources and influence to the long-term health of community members. This could extend from job creation, safe housing, access to health care, and affordable food to business partnerships and loans.

The commodification of health care services in the United States is contrary to the notion of health as a human right. The bottom lines of health systems are usually discussed in dollars and cents, not in terms of health and justice. But the possibilities here are endless. Health care institutions working in pragmatic solidarity with the members of their neighboring community can create opportunities to improve health by addressing the social and structural conditions outside their doors.

Whether these institutional efforts can be large enough, serious enough, or deep enough to overcome a century of social and economic policies that have entrenched poverty and misery in so many neighborhoods remains to be seen. At the very least, though, there is institutional awareness that until the structural causes of mortality are addressed, health equity cannot be achieved. When a health system chooses to become an anchor for community health and vitality, it is admitting that the elimination of poverty, hardship, and inequality is paramount to good health.

And it takes an activated, vocal community as well. As we've seen, the voice of community members is critically important to get health and civic institutions to focus on equity. In Chicago in the last few years, local health activists have been at the forefront of public demonstrations that have demanded the preservation of the public mental health system (unsuccessful), the preservation of access for the undocumented to transplant lists (partially successful), the creation of a trauma center on the South Side (successful), and the closing of an asthma-causing coal-fueled power plant (successful).[26]

What if the power and influence of health care systems combined with the experience of community leaders could be collectively focused on breaking down the structural barriers that have contributed to illness and premature mortality nationwide? Neighborhood by neighborhood, could we turn the tide on inequity and premature mortality?

Often I am asked why, in the face of so much evidence of a growing tide of human suffering, I remain hopeful. To witness, to speak and write about human misery and premature death, is a risky business indeed. I often face silence or uncomfortable avoidance when I raise these issues. I'll admit as well that it is difficult to face the despair of others without feeling despair myself at times. Writing and speaking about inequity makes me recalls memories and events I would rather sometimes leave unstirred. In my attempt to make an invisible America of poverty and pain visible, I may have scared some readers away. Or worse, I may have understated or soft-pedaled the magnitude of the problem and the difficulty of the solutions.

Social, economic, and racial inequities are wickedly complex problems that do not lend themselves to quick fixes or simple solutions. But I do remain optimistic that we can win. I am optimistic because the United States was born of slavery yet fought a civil war to end it. I am optimistic because the United States, having reshackled the black population with Jim Crow laws, a form of legal peonage, later outlawed this legalized discrimination in response to civil protests and rebellions. I am optimistic that as a result of the #BlackLivesMatter rebellions and the insights of writers like Michelle Alexander we will eventually overcome the oppression of mass imprisonment and other forms of structural racism.[27] I am optimistic because this is a country that gave women the right to vote after seventy years of protests and denial. I have seen my wife and daughter have opportunities during their lifetimes that were denied my mother and grandmother. I am optimistic because this is a country that gave people who love each other the right to marry anyone they want under the protection of the law.

Despite the long track record of structural violence in the United States, we have occasionally gotten it right for the betterment of all. Mostly I am optimistic because my practice of medicine has granted me the opportunity to witness the dignity and determination of patients like Windora who deserve more. My patients have given me so much in return and have asked so little. I am optimistic on their behalf. Health as a human right is not an abstract and distant notion. I am optimistic that when it comes to achieving health equity, after so many missteps, we will ultimately do the right thing. Martin Luther King Jr. once optimistically said, "The arc of the moral universe is long, but it bends toward justice."[28] I believe that is true, but only if we all bend the arc together.

ACKNOWLEDGMENTS

I could not have written this book were it not for the help of many others. The late Dr. Steven Whitman, a social epidemiologist and revolutionary, who throughout his adult life studied and battled the virulent effects of racism and other inequalities on health, was a great influence on the ideas I have expressed here. Steve was the director of the Sinai Urban Health Institute in Chicago and my dear friend. His work over three decades is prominently featured in this book.

I want to thank many student research assistants who aided the manuscript development. Gabriella "Ika" Kovacikova researched the work of Robert Sampson and other urban sociologists. That she also managed to train and then successfully swim the English Channel while working on the book was nothing short of amazing. Nevatha Mathialagan worked on the social underpinnings of natural disasters. Amy Isabelle contributed to the work on social cohesion and collective efficacy and to reference checking. Marieli Guzman worked with me on the problem of health care access for noncitizen residents of Chicago and on finding photos. Marycarmen Flores contributed to the section on health care for the undocumented, and she interviewed her aunt about the premature death of Marycarmen's first cousin Sarai, whose death at age 25 is highlighted in the book. Mira Bansal gave exquisite attention to detail regarding the figures and photos. Energy and passion for social justice and scholarship were evident in each of these students. All are pursuing health science careers.

This book would not have been completed without the considerable and incomparable help of my primary research associate and colleague, the indefatigable Kristen Pallok. Kristen volunteered for the four years it took to research and write the book. She conducted interviews and research, read and critiqued chapters in their earliest drafts, and helped with the manuscript development down to the finest detail. Kristen's contributions strengthened and sharpened the manuscript. That she has stuck with this project from its inception is a testament to her tenacity and passion for the subject matter. Kristen matriculated into Rush Medical College during this period and is well along her way of becoming a physician herself.

I must also acknowledge the wonderful support I received from Timothy Mennel, senior editor at the University of Chicago Press, whose skillful editing shaped the final manuscript into a book. His belief in this book has been invaluable. The whole team at University of Chicago Press has been nothing short of spectacular in their support of me during the publishing process. I also must acknowledge my literary agent, Susan Schulman, whose advice as the process unfolded has been both gracious and wise. My brother-in-law Stuart Grabler was an early reader, and his editing suggestions strengthened the manuscript considerably. My son Jonah Ansell contributed to conceptualizing the structure of the book and was the first to suggest the title *The Death Gap*. My daughter Leah Ansell and her husband Armeen Poor have always been ready participants in discussions of the subjects that became the basis for this book.

I must recognize the support and love of my wife and life partner, Dr. Paula Grabler, who has encouraged this project from its inception. She has tolerated my reading chapters out loud or discussing chapter ideas with her on long-distance runs. Her understanding of breast cancer mortality disparities contributed greatly to the chapter on health care inequalities. But her greatest contribution has been her unswerving belief in me and in the book over the years.

Finally, I want to thank my patients, who have allowed me a window into their lives and neighborhoods. I particularly want to thank the generosity of the Bradley family (a pseudonym) and especially

Windora, my patient, who opened her life and home to me. Through her openness and honesty, I was able to witness how inequality and structural violence took its toll on her, her family, and their community.

Chicago, July 2016

NOTES

Preface

1. Martin Luther King Jr., *Stride toward Freedom: The Montgomery Story* (London: Souvenir Press, 2011).
2. Milo Milton Quaife, *Chicago's Highways, Old and New, from Indian Trail to Motor Road* (Chicago: D.F. Keller, 1923).
3. Robert Crum, *Survey Identifies Health Issues in Six Chicago Communities, Leads to Targeted Interventions* (Princeton, NJ: Robert Wood Johnson Foundation, 2008).
4. Sabrina Tavernise and Albert Sun, "Same City, but Very Different Life Spans," *New York Times*, April 28, 2015.
5. Los Angeles County Department of Public Health, Office of Health Assessment and Epidemiology, "Life Expectancy in Los Angeles County: How Long Do We Live and Why? A Cities and Communities Report," July 2010.
6. Paul Galloway, "Gentle Giant of Skid Row," *Chicago Tribune*, June 14, 1987.
7. Ronald Kotulak, "State Mapping Plan for AIDS Epidemic," *Chicago Tribune*, December 8, 1985.
8. "Rush History," http://www.rush.edu/rumc/page-1134773754867.html, accessed July 8, 2013.
9. "North Lawndale History," Steans Family Foundation, http://www.steansfamily foundation.org/lawndale_history.shtml, accessed July 8, 2013.
10. "North Lawndale History," Lawndale Christian Health Center, http://www .lawndale.org/content/north-lawndale-history, accessed July 8, 2013.
11. "North Lawndale," Chicago Neighborhood Stabilization Program 2013, http:// www.chicagonsp.org/Our-neighborhoods/Neighborhoods-where-NSP-Chicago -has-acquired-properties/North-Lawndale.html, accessed July 8, 2013.
12. James Coates, "Riots Follow Killing of Martin Luther King Jr.," *Chicago Tribune*, April 5, 1968.
13. Gary Rivlin, "The Night Chicago Burned," *Chicago Reader*, August 25, 1988.
14. "North Lawndale: Faith Rewarded," Lawndale Christian Development Center, Local Initiatives Support Corporation, Chicago, May 2005.

15. "Western Electric Co," in *The Electronic Encyclopedia of Chicago* (Chicago: Chicago Historical Society, 2005).

16. "North Lawndale History," Steans Family Foundation.

17. Beryl Satter, *Family Properties: Race, Real Estate, and the Exploitation of Black Urban America* (New York: Macmillan, 2009).

18. Matthew Desmond, *Evicted: Poverty and Profit in the American City* (New York: Crown, 2016); Michelle Alexander, *The New Jim Crow: Mass Incarceration in the Age of Colorblindness* (New York: New Press, 2011).

Chapter 1

1. Paul Farmer, "On Suffering and Structural Violence: A View from Below," *Daedalus*, 1996, 261–83.

2. Douglas S. Massey, *Categorically Unequal: The American Stratification System* (New York: Russell Sage Foundation, 2008), xvi.

3. Donald Bartlett and James Steele. *The Betrayal of the American Dream* (New York: PublicAffairs, 2013).

4. Ibid.

5. Sylvia Allegretto,"One Step Up and Two Steps Back," *Berkeley Blog*, October 2, 2014, http://berkeleyblog.wpengine.com/wp-content/uploads/2014/10/BB2014.png.

6. Bartlett and Steele, *Betrayal of the American Dream*.

7. Organisation for Economic Control and Development (OECD), "Life Expectancy at Birth," 2016.

8. Paul Farmer, *Pathologies of Power: Health, Human Rights and the New War on the Poor* (Berkeley: University of California Press, 2003).

9. Paul Farmer, *Infections and Inequalities: The Modern Plagues* (Berkeley: University of California Press, 2001).

10. Bijou Hunt and Steve Whitman. "Black:White Health Disparities in the United States and Chicago: 1990–2010," *Journal of Racial and Ethnic Health Disparities* 2, no. 1 (2015): 93–100.

11. Dorothy Roberts, *Killing the Black Body: Race, Reproduction, and the Meaning of Liberty* (New York: Vintage, 2014).

12. Gina Kolata and Sarah Cohen, "Drug Overdoses Propel Rise in Mortality Rates of Young Whites," *New York Times*, January 16, 2016.

13. Anne Case and Angus Deaton, "Rising Morbidity and Mortality in Midlife among White Non-Hispanic Americans in the 21st Century," *Proceedings of the National Academy of Sciences of the United States of America* 112, no. 49 (2015): 15078–83.

14. Annie Lowrey, "Income Gap, Meet the Longevity Gap," *New York Times*, March 15, 2014.

15. Farmer, *Pathologies of Power*.

16. Groundspeak, "Louis Pasteur Memorial—Cook County Hospital, Chicago, IL—Statues of Historic Figures on Waymarking.com," http://www.waymarking.com/waymarks/WM3RPF, accessed December 10, 2013.

Chapter 2

1. H. Jack Geiger, "Why We Do What We Do," speech, Doctors for Global Health, August 2002, http://www.dghonline.org/content/what-we-do-and-why-we-do-it, accessed June 17, 2016.

2. US Geological Survey, "Earthquake Information for 2010," December 12, 2011, http://earthquake.usgs.gov/earthquakes/eqarchives/year/2010/.

3. US Geological Survey, "Historic Earthquakes," November 1, 2012, http://earth quake.usgs.gov/earthquakes/states/events/1989_10_18.php; "Comparison of the Bay Area Earthquakes: 1906 and 1989," in *San Andreas Fault*, 5–10 (US Geological Survey, 2005).

4. American Red Cross, "Disaster Preparedness in Haiti," March 2013, http://www .redcross.org/images/MEDIA_CustomProductCatalog/m17240223_Disaster _Preparedness_in_Haiti_01.pdf; Paul E. Weisenfeld, "Success and Challenges of the Haiti Earthquake Response: The Experience of USAID," *Emory International Law Review*, 2011, 1097–1120.

5. Lionel J. (Bo) Beaulieu and Deborah Tootle, *Helping Disadvantaged Populations Prepare for Disasters: Assessing the Efficacy of the Emergency Preparedness Demonstration Framework* (Mississippi State: Southern Rural Development Center, USDA, FEMA, and University of Arkansas, 2010).

6. Franklin W. Knight, *The Haitian Revolution* (Oxford: Oxford University Press, 2000); Paul Farmer, *Pathologies of Power: Health, Human Rights, and the New War on the Poor* (Berkeley: University of California Press, 2004).

7. Theodore Brown and Elizabeth Fee, "Rudolf Carl Virchow: Medical Scientist, Social Reformer, Role Model," *American Journal of Public Health*, 2006, 2104–5.

8. Salim Virani, A. N. Khan, and Eduardo de Marchena, "Takotsubo Cardiomyopathy, or Broken-Heart Syndrome," *Texas Heart Institute Journal*, 2007, 76–79.

9. Lawrence K. Altman, "Making the Right Call, Even in Death," *New York Times*, July 1, 2013.

10. R. Hanzlick, "Death Registration: History, Methods, and Legal Issues." *Journal of Forensic Sciences*, 1997, 265–69.

11. US Central Intelligence Agency, "Country Comparison: Life Expectancy at Birth," in *The World Factbook 2013–14* (Washington, DC: Central Intelligence Agency, 2013).

12. Thomas Kirkwood, "A System Look at an Old Problem," *Nature*, 2008, 644–47.

13. Sarah Burd-Sharps, Kristen Lewis, and Eduardo Borges Martins, *A Portrait of Mississippi: Mississippi Human Development Report*, American Human Development Project, 2009.

14. US Centers for Disease Control and Prevention, *Healthy People 2000 Final Review* (Hyattsville, MD: CDCP, 2001), and *Healthy People 2010 Final Review* (Atlanta: US Department of Health and Human Services, 2010).

15. Robert Pear, "Gap in Life Expectancy Widens for the Nation," *New York Times*, March 23, 2008; C. J. L. Murray, S. C. Kulkarni, C. Michaud, and N. Tomijima,

"Eight Americas: Investigating Mortality Disparities across Races, Countries, and Race—Counties in the United States." *PLoS Medicine*, 2006; UN Development Programme, *Human Development Reports: About Human Development, 2013*, http://hdr.undp.org/en/humandev/, accessed July 23, 2013; Burd-Sharps, Lewis, and Borges Martins, *Portrait of Mississippi*.

16. Hilary Waldron, "Trends in Mortality Differentials and Life Expectancy for Male Social Security–Covered Workers, by Average Relative Earnings," US Social Security Administration Office of Policy, 2007; Congressional Budget Office, *Growing Disparities in Life Expectancy*, Economic and Budget Issue Brief, Congress of the United States, 2008.

17. Colin McCord and Harold Freeman, "Excess Mortality in Harlem," *New England Journal of Medicine*, 1990, 1606–7.

18. Jennifer M. Orsi, Helen Margellos-Anast, and Steven Whitman, "Black-White Health Disparities in the United States and Chicago: A 15-Year Progress Analysis," *American Journal of Public Health*, 2010, 349–56; Steven Whitman, Ami Shah, and Maureen R. Benjamins, *Urban Health: Combating Disparities with Local Data* (Oxford: Oxford University Press, 2011).

19. Ibid.

20. Nancy Krieger et al., "The Fall and Rise of US Inequities in Premature Mortality: 1960–2002," *PLoS Medicine*, 2008.

21. A.T. Geronimus, J. Bound, and C. G. Colen, "Excess Black Mortality in the United States and in Select Black or White High-Poverty Areas." *American Journal of Public Health*, 2011, 720–29.

22. National Center for Health Statistics, *Health, United States, 2015: With Special Feature on Racial and Ethnic Health Disparities* (Hyattsville, MD, NCHS, 2016).

23. Geronimus, Bound, and Colen, "Excess Black Mortality."

24. Ibid.

Chapter 3

1. Lyndon B. Johnson, speech delivered at Howard University, June 4, 1965, http://www.lbjlib.utexas.edu/johnson/archives.hom/650604.

2. "Sociologist, with a Grand Agenda, W. E. B. Du Bois," African American Registry, http://www.aaregistry.org/historic_events/view/sociologist-grand-agenda-web-du -bois, accessed October 26, 2013; W. E. B. Du Bois and Isabel Eton. *The Philadelphia Negro: A Social Study* (Boston: Ginn, 1899).

3. Douglas S. Massey, "The Age of Extremes: Concentrated Affluence and Poverty in the Twenty-First Century," *Demography* 33, no. 4 (1996): 395–412.

4. Nicholas Lemann, *The Promised Land: The Great Black Migration and How It Changed America.* (New York: Alfred A. Knopf, 1991).

5. Du Bois and Eton, *The Philadelphia Negro*; Douglas S. Massey and Nancy A. Denton, *American Apartheid: Segregation and the Making of the Underclass* (Cambridge, MA: Harvard University Press, 1993).

6. L. P. Boustan, "Racial Residential Segregation in American Cities," in *Oxford Hand-*

NOTES TO PAGES 28–32 * 199

book of Urban Economics and Planning, ed. Nancy Brooks, Kieran Bonaghy, and Gerrit-Jan Knaap (New York: Oxford University Press, 2011), 318–39; Beryl Satter, *Family Properties: Race, Real Estate, and the Exploitation of Black Urban America* (New York: Henry Holt, 2009).

7. John McKnight, phone interview by author and Kristen Pallok, Chicago, October 22, 2013.

8. Bill Dedman, "The Color of Money: Southside Treated like Banks' Stepchild," *Atlanta Journal-Constitution*, May 2, 1988.

9. Ibid.

10. Ibid.

11. D. Bradford Hunt, "Redlining," in *The Encyclopedia of Chicago*, ed. James R. Grossman, Ann Durkin Keating, and Janice L. Reiff (Chicago: University of Chicago Press, 2005), http://www.encyclopedia.chicagohistory.org/pages/1050.html.

12. McKnight interview, October 22, 2013.

13. Satter, *Family Properties*.

14. Karl Taeuber, Center for Demography and Ecology University of Wisconsin–Madison, "Residence and Race: 1619 to 2019 CDE Working Paper 88–19," last modified 1988, http://www.ssc.wisc.edu/cde/cdewp/88–19.pdf, accessed November 21, 2013.

15. George Lipsitz, *The Possessive Investment in Whiteness* (Philadelphia: Temple University Press, 2006).

16. Satter, *Family Properties*; McKnight interview, October 22, 2013.

17. Satter, *Family Properties*; William Julius Wilson, *When Work Disappears: The World of the New Urban Poor* (New York: Random House, 1996).

18. Robert J. Sampson, *Great American City: Chicago and the Enduring Neighborhood Effect* (Chicago: University of Chicago Press, 2012).

19. "Chicago Housing Called Midwest's Most Segregated," *Chicago Sun Times*, December 7, 1962, 38.

20. John Kasarda and Allan Parnell, *Third World Cities: Problems, Policies and Prospects* (Newbury Park, CA: Sage, 1992).

21. Steve Bogira, "A Dream Unrealized for African-Americans in Chicago," *Chicago Reader*, last modified August 21, 2013, http://www.chicagoreader.com/chicago/african-american-percentage-poverty-unemployment-schools-segregation/Content?oid=10703562, accessed November 21, 2013; Sinai Urban Health Institute, *Chicago Community Health Profile: South Lawndale* (Chicago: Sinai Health System, 2001).

22. Wilson, *When Work Disappears*.

23. Kasarda and Parnell, *Third World Cities*; Massey and Denton, *American Apartheid*.

24. Bogira, "Dream Unrealized for African-Americans in Chicago."

25. Lipsitz, *Possessive Investment in Whiteness*.

26. Ibid.

27. National Interstate and Defense Highways Act (1956), Our Documents, http://www.ourdocuments.gov/doc.php?flash=true&doc=88, accessed October 24, 2013.

28. Adam Cohen and Elizabeth Taylor, *American Pharaoh: Mayor Richard J. Daley— His Battle for Chicago and the Nation* (New York: Little, Brown, 2000).

29. R. L. Schiff et al., "Transfers to a Public Hospital. A Prospective Study of 467 Patients," *New England Journal of Medicine*, no. 9 (1986): 552–57.

30. Massey, "Age of Extremes"; Sampson, *Great American City*.

31. Massey, "Age of Extremes."

32. Satter, *Family Properties*.

33. Mark Seitles, "The Perpetuation of Residential Racial Segregation in America: Historical Discrimination, Modern Forms of Exclusion, and Inclusionary Remedies," *Journal of Land Use and Environmental Law*, 1996.

34. Massey and Denton, *American Apartheid*.

35. Sampson, *Great American City*.

36. William H. Frey, "A Snapshot of Race in America's Neighborhoods." *Atlantic*, June 11, 2015.

37. "500 Top Foreclosure Zip Codes," CNNMoney, June 19, 2007, http://money.cnn.com/2007/06/19/real_estate/500_top_foreclosure_zip_codes/, accessed February 22, 2014.

38. Kristopher Gerardi and Paul Willen, "The Mortgage Meltdown, the Economy and Public Policy Subprime Mortages, Foreclosures, and Urban Neighborhoods," *B.E. Journal of Economic Analysis and Policy* 9, no. 3 (2009): 1–35.

39. Boustan, "Racial Residential Segregation in American Cities"; Seitles, "Perpetuation of Residential Racial Segregation in America."

40. Bogira, "Dream Unrealized for African-Americans in Chicago."

41. Patrick Sharkey, *Stuck in Place: Urban Neighborhoods and the End of Progress toward Racial Equality* (Chicago: University of Chicago Press, 2013).

42. Steven Whitman, interview by author, Chicago, 2013.

43. Whitman interview; Colin McCord and Harold P. Freeman, "Excess Mortality in Harlem," *New England Journal of Medicine* 322 (1990): 173–77.

44. "History: Provident Hospital," Provident Foundation, http://www.providentfoundation.org/history/, accessed October 24, 2013; Gabriel Spitzer, "Cook County Hospitals Cut Nurses, Some Ambulance Service," WBEZ radio, last modified February 15, 2011, http://www.wbez.org/story/cook-county/cook-county-hospitals-cut-nurses-some-ambulance-service, accessed November 21, 2013.

45. World Bank, "Life Expectancy at Birth," http://data.worldbank.org/indicator/SP.DYN.LE00.IN?order=wbapi_data_value_2013+wbapi_data_value&sort=asc, accessed May 30, 2016.

46. Robert Wood Johnson Foundation, *Commission to Build a Healthier America— City Maps*, 2013, http://www.rwjf.org/en/about-rwjf/newsroom/features-and-articles/commission/resources/city-maps.html, accessed July 26, 2013.

47. Christopher J. L. Murray et al., "Eight Americas: Investigating Mortality Disparities across Races, Counties, and Race-Counties in the United States." *PLOS Medicine* 3, no. 9 (2006): 1513–24.

48. Robert Wood Johnson Foundation. *Commission to Build a Healthier America— City Maps*.

49. Murray, "Eight Americas."

50. "The Pine Ridge Reservation Demographics, 2009," Red Cloud Indian School, www.redcloudschool.org/history/072409_PineRidge_FactSheet.pdf.

51. Gina Kolata and Sarah Cohen, "Drug Overdoses Propel Rise in Mortality Rates of Young Whites," *New York Times*, January 16, 2016.

52. Ibid.

53. Ibid.

54. Angus Deaton, "On Death and Money: History, Facts, and Explanations," *Journal of the American Medical Association (JAMA)*, 2016.

55. Raj Chetty et al., "The Association between Income and Life Expectancy in the United States, 2001–2014," *JAMA*, 2016.

56. "Segregation: Dissimilarity Indices," CensusScope, http://www.censusscope.org /index.html, accessed July 26, 2013.

57. Theodore R. Johnson, "What if Black America Were a Country?" *Atlantic*, October 14, 2014, http://www.theatlantic.com/international/archive/2014/10/what-if -black-america-were-a-country/380953/.

58. "Martin Luther King I Have a Dream Speech—American Rhetoric," Estate of Dr. Martin Luther King Jr., http://www.americanrhetoric.com/speeches/mlk ihaveadream.htm, accessed October 24, 2013.

Chapter 4

1. Kerner Commisssion and Tom Wicker, *Report of the National Advisory Commission on Civil Disorders* (New York: Bantam Books, 1968).

2. Latino communities in the US are often places of concentrated poverty *and* high life expectancy—a situation known as the "Hispanic Paradox." Speculation is that those who can migrate over long distances may be healthier than those who stay behind. But really, no one knows the reasons.

3. Donald Bartlett and James Steele, *The Betrayal of the American Dream* (New York: Public Affairs, 2013).

4. Ibid.

5. Ibid.

6. G. William Domhoff, "Wealth, Income, and Power," *Who Rules America?*, last modified February 2013, http://www2.ucsc.edu/whorulesamerica/power/wealth .html.

7. Neal Gabler, "The Secret Shame of Middle Class Americans," *Atlantic*, May 2016.

8. Bartlett and Steele, *Betrayal of the American Dream*.

9. Kristen Weir, "Closing the Health-Wealth Gap," *American Psychological Association* 44, no. 9 (2013): 36.

10. Robert Sampson and Stephen W. Raudenbush, "Neighborhood Stigma and the Perception of Disorder," *Focus* 24, no. 1 (2005): 7–11.

11. "The American Millstone," *Chicago Tribune*, 1986.

12. Sinai Urban Health Institute, *Chicago Community Health Profile: North Lawndale* (Chicago: Sinai Health System, 2001).

13. "American Millstone."

14. William I. Thomas and Florian Znaniecki, *The Polish Peasant in Europe and America: Monograph of an Immigrant Group* (Boston: Gorham, 1918); E. Franklin Frazier, *The Negro Family in Chicago* (Chicago: University of Chicago Press, 1932); Robert J. Sampson, *Great American City: Chicago and the Enduring Neighborhood Effect* (Chicago: University of Chicago Press, 2012); Sinai Urban Health Institute, *Chicago Community Health Profile: South Lawndale* (Chicago: Sinai Health System, 2001); Roger A. Salerno, *Louis Wirth: A Bio-Bibliography* (Santa Barbara, CA: Greenwood, 1987).

15. Albert Hunter, "Symbols of Incivility: Social Disorder and Fear of Crime in Urban Neighborhoods," Northwestern University Center for Urban Affairs, November 1978.

16. Sampson, *Great American City*; George Kelling and James Q. Wilson, "Broken Windows," *Atlantic*, March 1, 1982.

17. Kelling and Wilson, "Broken Windows."

18. Sampson, *Great American City*.

19. Daniel Brook, "The Cracks in 'Broken Window,'" *Boston Globe*, February 19, 2006.

20. Ken Auletta, "Fixing Broken Windows," *New Yorker*, September 7, 2015.

21. Bernard E. Harcourt and Jens Ludwig, "Broken Windows: New Evidence from New York City and a Five-City Social Experiment," University of Chicago Public Law and Legal Theory Working Paper 93 (2005).

22. Sampson, *Great American City*.

23. Ibid.

24. Chad Boutin, "Snap Judgments Decide a Face's Character, Psychologist Finds," *News at Princeton*, August 22, 2006, http://www.princeton.edu/main/news /archive/S15/62/69K40/index.xml?section=topstories; Malcolm Gladwell, *Blink: The Power of Thinking without Thinking* (New York: Little, Brown, 2005).

25. Robert J. Sampson, "Seeing Disorder: Neighborhood Stigma and the Social Construction of 'Broken Windows,'" *Social Psychology Quarterly* 67, no. 4 (2004): 319–42.

26. Shankar Vedantam, *The Hidden Brain* (New York: Spiegel and Grau, 2010).

27. J. Correll, "The Police Officer's Dilemma: Using Ethnicity to Disambiguate Potentially Threatening Individuals," *Journal of Personality and Social Psychology* 83, no. 6 (2002): 1314–29.

28. "Ask the Expert Robert J. Sampson." *Advanced Study in the Behavioral Sciences at Stanford University*, June 29, 2012.

29. Robert J. Sampson, Chicago Project, Harvard University, http://scholar.harvard .edu/sampson/content/chicago-project-phdcn-0, accessed August 2, 2013.

30. Sampson, *Great American City*.

31. Lawrence Bobo, *Racial Attitudes and Relations at the Close of the 20th Century*, ed. N. J. Smelser, W.,G. Wilson, and F. Mitchell (Washington, DC: National Academy Press, 2001).

32. "American Millstone."

33. Sampson, *Great American City*.

34. Lincoln Quillian and Devah Pager, "Black Neighbors, Higher Crime? The Role of

Racial Stereotypes in Evaluations of Neighborhood Crime," *American Journal of Sociology*, 2001, 717–67.

35. Douglas S. Massey and Nancy A. Denton, *American Apartheid: Segregation and the Making of the Underclass* (Cambridge, MA: Harvard University Press, 1993).

36. Sampson, *Great American City*; Robert Wood Johnson Foundation, *Commision to Build a Healthier America—City Maps*, 2013, http://www.rwjf.org/en/about-rwjf /newsroom/features-and-articles/Commission/resources/city-maps.html, accessed July 26, 2013.

37. Robert C. Embry Jr., "To Improve Outcomes for Poor Kids, Let Them Move to the Suburbs," *Baltimore Sun*, February 9. 2011, http://articles.baltimoresun.com/2011 –02–09/news/bs-ed-poor-children-20110209_1_poor-children-low-income -children-public-housing.

38. Sampson, *Great American City*; Lincoln Quillian, *Migration and the Maintenance of Racial Segregation* (Madison: Center for Demography and Ecology, University of Wisconsin, 1998).

39. Sampson, *Great American City*.

Chapter 5

1. Greg Johnson, "Q and A with Dorothy Roberts," *Penn Current*, October 16, 2014, https://penncurrent.upenn.edu/2014–10–16/interviews/qa-dorothy-roberts, ac- cessed June 17, 2014.

2. Quamrul Ashraf and Oded Galor, "The 'Out of Africa; Hypothesis, Human Genetic Diversity, and Comparative Economic Development," *American Economic Review* 103, no. 1 (2013).

3. "Doomed to Failure by 'Poverty Gene,'" *Scotsman*, May 21, 2006, http://www.scots man.com/news/health/doomed-to-failure-by-poverty-gene-1-1412072, accessed May 6, 2014.

4. Kirsten Stewart, "Poor, Uninsured Women Prone to Late-Stage Breast Cancer, Says U. of Utah Study," *Salt Lake Tribune*, March 5, 2013, http://www.sltrib.com/sltrib /news/55952915–78/cancer-late-utah-health.html.csp.

5. Caitlin Dickerson, "Secret World War II Chemical Experiments Tested Troops by Race," NPR, June 22, 2015. http://www.npr.org/2015/06/22/415194765/u-s-troops -tested-by-race-in-secret-world-war-ii-chemical-experiments.

6. C. E. Grim and M. Robinson, "Commentary: Salt, Slavery, and Survival— Hypertension in the African Diaspora," *Epidemiology* 14, no. 1 (2003): 120–22.

7. Jay S. Kaufman and Susan A. Hall, "The Slavery Hypertension Hypothesis: Dis- semination and Appeal of a Modern Race Theory," *Epidemiology* 14, no. 1 (2003): 111–18; "Best of Oprah: Ask Dr. Oz," *Oprah Winfrey Show*, dir. Joseph C. Terry, April 26, 2007.

8. Dorothy Roberts, *Fatal Invention: How Science, Politics and Big-Business Re-create Race in the Twenty-First Century* (New York: New Press, 2011), 26; Nicolas Wade, "For Genome Mappers, the Tricky Terrain of Race Requires Some Careful Navigat- ing," *New York Times*, July 20, 2001, http://www.nytimes.com/2001/07/20/us/for

-genome-mappers-the-tricky-terrain-of-race-requires-some-careful-navigating
.html.

9. Marla Paul, "Childhood Asthma Varies by Neighborhood," Northwestern University, February 19, 2008. http://www.northwestern.edu/newscenter/stories/2008/02/asthma.html.

10. "Chicago Asthma Epidemic: The Status of Asthma in Chicago," *Respiratory Health Association of Chicago*, 2007.

11. Matthew Blake, "Little Village Residents Cheer Coal Plant Closings," *Progress Illinois*, March 1, 2012, http://www.progressillinois.com/posts/content/2012/02/29/pilsen-little-village-residents-cheer-coal-plant-shut-down.

12. Sara Ganim and Lihn Tran, "How Tap Water Became Toxic in Flint, Michigan." CNN, January 13, 2016, http://edition.cnn.com/2016/01/11/health/toxic-tap-water-flint-michigan/.

13. "Flint City, Michigan," *QuickFacts*, US Census Bureau, 2014.

14. Nicholas Kristof, "America Is Flint," *New York Times*, February 6, 2016.

15. Marcia Angell, *The Truth about the Drug Companies* (New York: Random House, 2004); Steve Morgan and Jae Kennedy. *Prescription Drug Accessibility and Affordability in the United States and Abroad*, Commonwealth Fund1408:89, June 2010.

16. Another line of argument is that the FDA should not have approved it at all. The component medications have been freely available as separate compounds for years. By achieving FDA approval, the patent on the two drugs was extended to 2020. And there are better and less expensive medications already on the market.

17. D. E. Roberts, "What's Wrong with Race-Based Medicine? Genes, Drugs, and Health Disparities," *Minnesota Journal of Law, Science and Technology* 12, no. 1 (2011): 1–21.

18. Erin Wigger, "The Whitehall Study," Unhealthy Work: Center for Social Epidemiology, June 22, 2011, http://unhealthywork.org/classic-studies/the-whitehall-study/.

19. Angus Deaton, "On Death and Money: History, Facts, and Explanations," *JAMA*, 2016.

20. Nancy Krieger, "Embodiment: A Conceptual Glossary for Epidemiology," *Journal for Epidemiology and Community Health* 59 (2005): 350–55.

21. Sarah Mustillo et al., "Self-Reported Feelings of Racial Discrimination and Black-White Differences in Preterm and Low-Birthweight Deliveries: The CARDIA Study," *American Journal of Public Health* 94, no. 12 (2004): 2125–31.

22. Angus Deaton, "Policy Implications of the Gradient of Health and Wealth," *Health Affairs* 21, no. 2 (2002): 13–30.

23. John Lynch et al., "Is Income Inequality a Determinant of Population Health? Part 1: A Systematic Review," *Milbank Quarterly* 82, no. 1 (2004): 5–99; John Lynch et al., "Is Income Inequality a Determinant of Population Health? Part 2: US National and Regional Trends in Income Inequality and Age- and Cause-Specific Mortality," *Milbank Quarterly* 82, no. 2 (2004): 355–400.

24. Angus Deaton, *The Great Escape: Health, Wealth, and the Origins of Inequality* (Princeton, NJ: Princeton University Press, 2013).

25. Ibid.

26. Nancy Krieger, "Methods for the Scientific Study of Discrimination and Health: An Ecosocial Approach," *American Journal of Public Health* 102, no. 5 (2012): 936–44; Raj Chetty et al., "The Association between Income and Life Expectancy in the United States, 2001–2014," *JAMA*, 2016.

27. Chetty et al., "Association between Income and Life Expectancy."

28. Arline Geronimus, "Do US Black Women Experience Stress-Related Accelerated Biological Aging? A Novel Theory and First Population-Based Test of Black-White Difference in Telomere Length," *Human Nature* 21, no. 1 (2010): 19–38; Jama L. Purser, "Geographical Segregation and IL-6: A Marker of Chronic Inflammation in Older Adults," *Biomark Med* 2, no. 4 (2008): 335–48; John S. Yudkin, "Inflammation, Obesity, Stress and Coronary Heart Disease: Is Interleukin-6 the Link?" *Atherosclerosis* 148, no. 2 (2000): 209–14.

29. P. H. Black, "The Inflammatory Response Is an Integral Part of the Stress Response: Implications for Atherosclerosis, Insulin Resistance, Type II Diabetes and Metabolic Syndrome X," *Brain Behavior and Immunity* 17, no. 5 (2003): 350–64.

30. Ibid.; Bruce McEwen and Teresa Seeman, "Allostatic Load and Allostasis," University of California, San Francisco, August 2009, http://www.macses.ucsf.edu /research/allostatic/allostatic.php, accessed October 21, 2016.

31. Jeongok G. Logan, "Allostasis and Allostatic Load: Expanding the Discourse on Stress and Cardiovascular Disease," *Journal of Clinical Nursing* 17, no. 7b (2008): 201–8.

32. Black, "Inflammatory Response Is an Integral Part of the Stress Response."

33. R. M. Meyer, "A Ghrelin–Growth Hormone Axis Drives Stress-Induced Vulnerability to Enhanced Fear," *Molecular Psychiatry*, 2013, 1–11; Zachary R. Patterson, "Ghrelin—The Defender of Fat in the Face of Stress: Implications in Obesity Treatment" (PhD diss., Carleton University, 2013).

34. McEwen, *MacArthur*; Patterson, "Ghrelin."

35. Purser, "Geographical Segregation and IL-6"; Brian K. Finch, "Neighborhood Effects on Health: Concentrated Advantage and Disadvantage," *Health Place* 16, no. 5 (2010): 1058–60.

36. Logan, "Allostasis and Allostatic Load"; Yudkin, "Inflammation, Obesity, Stress and Coronary Heart Disease."

37. D. L. van den Hove, "Maternal Stress-Induced Reduction in Birth Weight as a Marker for Adult Affective state," *Frontiers in Bioscience* 1, no. 2 (2010): 43–46.

38. James W. Collins Jr., "African-American Mothers' Perception of Their Residential Environment, Stressful Life Events, and Very Low Birthweight," *Epidemiology* 9, no. 3 (1998): 286–89.

39. Robert S. Lindsay, "Inhibition of 11β-Hydroxysteroid Dehydrogenase in Pregnant Rats and the Programming of Blood Pressure in the Offspring," *Hypertension* 27 (1996): 1200–1204; Keith M. Godfrey, "Fetal Nutrition and Adult Disease," *American Journal of Clinical Nutrition* 71, no. 5 (2000): 1344s–52s; D. J. Barker, "Growth In Utero, Blood Pressure in Childhood and Adult Life, and Mortality from Cardiovascular Disease," *British Journal of Medicine* 298, no. 6673 (1989): 564–67.

40. Nancy E. Reichman, "Low Birth Weight and School Readiness," *Future of Children* 15, no. 1 (2005): 91–116.

41. Richard J. David, "Differing Birth Weight among Infants of U.S.-Born Blacks, African-Born Blacks, and U.S.-Born Whites," *New England Journal of Medicine* 337 (1997): 1209–14.

42. Mustillo et al., "Self-Reported Experiences of Racial Discrimination."

43. Elizabeth H. Blackburn, "Maternal Psychosocial Stress during Pregnancy Is Associated with Newborn Leukocyte Telomere Length," *American Journal of Obstetrics and Gynecology* 208, no. 2 (2013): 134.e1–e7; A. O'Donovan, "Stress Appraisals and Cellular Aging: A Key Role for Anticipatory Threat in the Relationship between Psychological Stress and Telomere Length," *Brain Behavior and Immunity* 26, no. 4 (2012): 573–79; Elissa S. Epel, "Accelerated Telomere Shortening in Response to Life Stress," *PNAS* 101, no. 49 (2004): 17,312–15.

44. Epel, "Accelerated Telomere Shortening in Response to Life Stress."

45. Geronimus, "Do US Black Women Experience Stress-Related Accelerated Biological Aging?"

46. Dellara F. Terry, "Association of Longer Telomeres with Better Health in Centenarians," *Journals of Gerontology Series A: Biological Sciences and Medical Sciences* 63, no. 8 (2010): 809–12.

47. Erik Eckholm, "Trying to Explain a Drop in Infant Mortality," *New York Times*, November 27, 2009.

48. Thomas Schlenker, "The Effect of Prenatal Support on Birth Outcomes in an Urban Midwestern County," *Western Journal of Medicine* 111, no. 6 (2012): 267–73.

49. Eckholm, "Trying to Explain a Drop in Infant Mortality."

50. Schlenker, "Effect of Prenatal Support on Birth Outcomes in an Urban Midwestern County"; David Wahlberg, "Dane County's Black-White Infant Mortality Gap Continues," *Wisconsin State Journal*, April 13, 2014.

51. Patrick Sharkey, *Stuck in Place: Urban Neighborhoods and the End of Progress toward Racial Equality* (Chicago: University of Chicago Press, 2013).

Chapter 6

1. Rex Taylor and Annelie Rieger, "Rudolf Virchow on the Typhus Epidemic in Upper Silesia: An Introduction and Translation," *Sociology of Health and Illness* 6, no. 2 (1984): 201–17.

2. Eric Klinenberg, *Heat Wave: A Social Autopsy of Disaster in Chicago* (Chicago: University of Chicago Press, 2002).

3. Ben Grove, "Morgue Tries to Keep Up with Heat Wave," *Chicago Tribune*, July 17, 1995, http://articles.chicagotribune.com/1995–07–17/news/9507170105_1_heat-wave-morgue-workers-medical-examiner.

4. Mike Thomas, "Heat Wave: An Oral History," *Chicago Magazine*, June 29, 2015.

5. Ibid.

6. Steve Whitman, interview by Darlene Oliver, unpublished transcript, April 26, 2012.

7. Much of his detective work became the basis for a best-selling book by Eric Klinenberg, *Heat Wave: A Social Autopsy of Disaster in Chicago* (Chicago: University of Chicago Press, 2002).

8. Mary Gail Snyder, "It Didn't Begin with Katrina," *National Housing Institute* 143 (September/October 2005), http://www.nhi.org/online/issues/143/beforekatrina.html.

9. Philip Locker, "Poor, Black, and Left to Die: What Hurricane Katrina Shows about American Capitalism," *CWI Reporters*, September 18, 2005.

10. "FEMA Chief: Victims Bear Some Responsibility." CNN.com, September 1, 2005, http://www.cnn.com/2005/WEATHER/09/01/katrina.fema.brown/.

11. Nicole M. Stephens et al., "Why Did They 'Choose' to Stay? Perspectives of Hurricane Katrina Observers and Survivors," *Psychological Science* 20, no. 7 (2009):878–86.

12. Jennifer Pangyanszki, "Three Days of Death, Despair and Survival," CNN, September 9, 2005.

13. Robert E. Pierre and Paul Farhi, "'Refugee': A Word of Trouble," *Washington Post*, September 7, 2005, http://www.washingtonpost.com/wp-dyn/content/article/2005/09/06/AR2005090601896.html.

14. Joan Brunkard, Gonza Namulanda, and Raoul Ratard, "Hurricane Katrina Deaths, Louisiana, 2005," *Disaster Mediccine and Public Health Preparedness* 2, no 4 (2008): 215.

Chapter 7

1. Michelle Alexander. *The New Jim Crow: Mass Incarceration in the Age of Colorblindness* (New York: New Press, 2010).

2. The most thorough and damning assessment of this racist system is Alexander, *New Jim Crow*.

3. Evan Osnos, "Father Mike," *New Yorker*, February 29, 2016.

4. Justin Wolfers, David Leonhardt, and Kevin Quealy, "1.5 Million Missing Black Men," *New York Times*, April 20, 2015, http://www.nytimes.com/interactive/2015/04/20/upshot/missing-black-men.html?_r=1.

5. Ibid.

6. John Blake, "'Lord of the Flies' Comes to Baltimore," CNN, May 4, 2015, http://edition.cnn.com/2015/05/02/us/lord-of-the-flies-baltimore/.

7. Christopher J. Lyons and Becky Pettit, "Compounded Disadvantage: Race, Incarceration, and Wage Growth," *Social Problems* 58, no. 2 (2011): 257–80.

8. Ibid.

9. Peter Wagner, "Tracking State Prison Growth in 50 States," *Prison Policy Institute*, May 28, 2014, http://www.prisonpolicy.org/reports/overtime.html.

10. Associated Press, "Report: 7 Million Americans in Justice System," Nbcnews.com, November 30, 2006, http://www.nbcnews.com/id/15960666/ns/us_news-crime_and_courts/t/report-million-americans-justice-system/.

11. Bruce Jake, "Incarceration Gap Widens between Blacks and Whites," *Pew Research Center*, September 6, 2013, http://www.pewresearch.org/fact-tank/2013/09/06 /incarceration-gap-between-whites-and-blacks-widens/.

12. Inimai M. Chettiar, "The Many Causes of America's Decline in Crime," *Atlantic*, February 11, 2015, http://www.theatlantic.com/politics/archive/2015/02/the-many -causes-of-americas-decline-in-crime/385364/; Olivia Roeder, Lauren-Brooke Eisen, and Julia Bowling, "What Caused the Crime Decline?" Brennan Center for Justice, February 12, 2015; Todd R. Clear, *Imprisoning Communities: How Mass Incarceration Makes Disadvantaged Neighborhoods Worse* (Oxford: Oxford University Press, 2007).

13. Steve Whitman, "The Crime of Black Imprisonment," *Chicago Tribune*, May 28, 1987.

14. Alexander, *New Jim Crow*.

15. Dora M. Durmont, "Public Health and the Epidemic of Incarceration," *Annual Review of Public Health* 33 (2012): 325–39.

16. Doris J. James and Lauren E. Glaze, "Mental Health Problems of Prison and Jail Inmates," US Department of Justice, September 2006.

17. "NRRC Facts & Trends," CSG Justice Center, https://csgjusticecenter.org/nrrc /facts-and-trends/, accessed April 25, 2016.

18. Laura M. Maruschak and Marcus Berzofsky, "Medical Problems of State and Federal Prisoners and Jail Inmates, 2011–12," US Department of Justice, February 2015.

19. Margaret Noonan, Harley Rohloff, and Scott Ginder, "Mortality in Local Jails and State Prisons, 2003–2013—Statistical Tables," US Department of Justice, August 2015.

20. Committee on International Human Rights, "Supermax Confinement in U.S. Prisons," New York City Bar Association, September 2011.

21. "Solitary Confinement Should Be Banned in Most Cases, UN Expert Says," UN News Centre, October 18, 2011, https://www.un.org/apps/news/story.asp?NewsID =40097.

22. Ingrid A. Binsanger et al., "Release from Prison—A High Risk of Death for Former Inmates," *New England Journal of Medicine* 356, no. 2 (2007): 157–65.

23. Christopher Wildeman, Hedwig Lee, and Megan Comfort, "A New Vulnerable Population? The Health of Female Partners of Men Recently Released from Prison," *Women's Health Issues* 23, no. 6 (2013).

24. Judith Graham, "Virulent Bacteria Hits Poor," *Chicago Tribune*, March 29, 2007, http://articles.chicagotribune.com/2007–05–29/news/0705280339_1_mrsa-hospital -acquired-staph-infections.

25. "FAQs about Children of Prisoners," Prison Fellowship, https://www.prisonfellow ship.org/resources/training-resources/family/ministry-basics/faqs-about-children -of-prisoners/, accessed April 24, 2016.

26. Alex Kotlowitz, *There Are No Children Here* (New York: Anchor Books, 1992), x.

27. Fyodor Dostoyevsky, *The House of the Dead*, trans. Constance Garnett (Vremya, 1862).

Chapter 8

1. Quoted in David Barsamian, *Louder Than Bombs: Interviews from the Progressive Magazine* (Boston: South End, 2004).
2. Julie Appleby, "FAQ: Obamacare and Coverage for Immigrants," *Kaiser Health News*, September 19, 2013. http://khn.org/news/health-care-immigrants/.
3. Ibid.
4. Leah Zallman et al., "Unauthorized Immigrants Prolong the Life of Medicare's Trust Fund," *Journal of General Internal Medicine* 31, no. 1 (2016): 122–27.
5. MaryCarmen Flores, interview with Victoria Rodriguez, unpublished transcript, August 5, 2014.
6. Ibid.
7. David Ansell et al., "When the Only Cure Is a Transplant," *Health Affairs* blog, February 21, 2014, http://healthaffairs.org/blog/2014/02/21/when-the-only-cure-is -a-transplant/.
8. Jakobi Williams, *From the Bullet to the Ballot: The Illinois Chapter of the Black Panther Party and Radical Coalition Politics in Chicago* (Chapel Hill: University of North Carolina Press, 2013), 196.

Chapter 9

1. Paul Farmer, *Infections and Inequalities: The Modern Plagues* (Berkeley: University of California Press, 2001).
2. David R. Williams and Pamela Braboy Jackson, "Social Sources of Racial Dispari-ties in Health," *Health Affairs* 24, no. 2 (2005): 325–34; James B. Kirby and Toshiko Kaneda, "Neighborhood Socioeconomic Disadvantage and Access to Health Care," *Journal of Health and Social Behavior* 46, no. 1 (2005): 15–31.
3. Allison L. Diamant et al., "Delays and Unmet Need for Health Care among Adult Primary Care Patients in a Restructured Urban Public Health System," *American Journal of Public Health* 94, no. 5 (2004): 783–89; John Z. Ayanian et al., "Unmet Health Needs of Uninsured Adults in the United States," *JAMA* 284, no. 16 (2000): 2061–69.
4. J. Michael McWilliams, Ellen Meara, Alan M. Zaslavsky, and John Z. Ayanian, "Use of Health Services by Previously Uninsured Medicare Beneficiaries," *New England Journal of Medicine* 357, no. 2 (2007): 143–53.
5. Elizabeth N. Chapman, Anna Kaatz, and Molly Carnes, "Physicians and Implicit Bias: How Doctors May Unwittingly Perpetuate Health Care Disparities," *Journal of General Internal Medicine* 28, no. 11 (2013): 1504–10.
6. American Cancer Society, *Cancer Facts and Figures 2015* (Atlanta: American Cancer Society; 2015).
7. Richard M. Elledge, Gary M. Clark, Gary C. Chamness, and C. Kent Osborne, "Tumor Biologic Factors and Breast Cancer Prognosis among White, Hispanic, and Black Women in the United States," *Journal of the National Cancer Institute* 86, no. 9 (1994): 705–12.

8. David Ansell, interview with Paula Grabler, August 13, 2015.

9. Edward A. Sickles, Dulcy E. Wolverton, and Katherine E. Dee, "Performance Parameters for Screening and Diagnostic Mammography: Specialist and General Radiologists 1," *Radiology* 224, no. 3 (2002): 861–69.

10. Metropolitan Chicago Breast Cancer Task Force, "Improving Quality and Reducing Disparities in Breast Cancer Mortality in Metropolitan Chicago," October 2007.

11. Garth H. Rauscher, Jenna A. Khan, Michael L. Berbaum, and Emily F. Conant, "Potentially Missed Detection with Screening Mammography: Does the Quality of Radiologists' Interpretation Vary by Patient Socioeconomic Advantage/Disadvantage?" *Annals of Epidemiology* 23, no. 4 (2013): 210–14; Yamile Molina, Abigail Silva, and Garth H. Rauscher, "Racial/Ethnic Disparities in Time to a Breast Cancer Diagnosis: The Mediating Effects of Health Care Facility Factors," *Medical Care* 53, no. 10 (2015): 872–78.

12. Rauscher et al., "Potentially Missed Detection With Screening Mammography.

13. "Where Are Chicago's Poor White Neighborhoods?," *Morning Edition*, WBEZ, August 12, 2015.

14. Jenna Khan et al., "Distribution of Mammography Facility and Census Tract Characteristics in Chicago," *Cancer Epidemiology Biomarkers and Prevention* 2012 (October 27, 2012), Proceedings of the Fifth AACR Conference on the Science of Cancer Health Disparities in Racial/ Ethnic Minorities and the Medically Underserved.

15. Jocelyn Hirschman, Steven Whitman, and David Ansell, "The Black:White Disparity in Breast Cancer Mortality: The Example of Chicago," *Cancer Causes and Control* 18, no. 3 (2007): 323–33.

16. Steven Whitman, David Ansell, Jennifer Orsi, and Teena Francois, "The Racial Disparity in Breast Cancer Mortality," *Journal of Community Health* 36, no. 4 (2011): 588–96.

17. Hirschman, Whitman, and Ansell, "Black:White Disparity in Breast Cancer Mortality."

18. Parisa Tehranifar et al., "Medical Advances and Racial/Ethnic Disparities in Cancer Survival," *Cancer Epidemiology Biomarkers and Prevention* 18, no. 10 (2009): 2701–8.

19. Tomi F. Akinyemiju et al., "Individual and Neighborhood Socioeconomic Status and Healthcare Resources in Relation to Black-White Breast Cancer Survival Disparities," *Journal of Cancer Epidemiology*, 2013.

20. Metropolitan Chicago Breast Cancer Task Force, "Improving Quality and Reducing Disparities in Breast Cancer Mortality in Metropolitan Chicago."

21. Whitman et al., "Racial Disparity in Breast Cancer Mortality."

22. Bijou R. Hunt, Steve Whitman, and Marc S. Hurlbert, "Increasing Black:White Disparities in Breast Cancer Mortality in the 50 Largest Cities in the United States," *Cancer Epidemiology* 38, no. 2 (2014): 118–23.

23. Ibid.

24. Ibid.

25. David Ansell et al., "A Community Effort to Reduce the Black/White Breast Cancer Mortality Disparity in Chicago," *Cancer Causes and Control* 20, no. 9 (2009): 1681–88.
26. Shane Trisch, "The Deadly Difference," *Chicago Magazine*, September 19, 2007.
27. Sunny Sea Gold, "Why Are So Many Black Women Dying of Breast Cancer?" *O, the Oprah Magazine*, October 2015.
28. Teena Francois-Blue, Katherine Tossas-Milligan, and Anne Marie Murphy, "Metropolitan Chicago Breast Cancer Task Force: How Far Have We Come? Improving Access to and Quality of Breast Health Services in Chicago," October 2014.
29. Gold, "Why Are So Many Black Women Dying of Breast Cancer?"
30. John Tierney, "A Shocking Test of Bias," *New York Times*, November 18, 2008.
31. Kevin A. Schulman et al., "The Effect of Race and Sex on Physicians' Recommendations for Cardiac Catheterization," *New England Journal of Medicine* 340 (1999): 618–26.
32. Brian Smedley, Adrienne Stith, and Alan Nelson, eds., "Unequal Treatment: Confronting Racial and Ethnic Disparities in Health Care: Report," Institute of Medicine, National Academies of Medicine, 2002.
33. Monica E. Peek et al., "Patient Trust in Physicians and Shared Decision-Making among African-Americans with Diabetes," *Health Communication* 28, no. 6 (2013): 616–23.
34. Stephanie E. Rogers et al., "Discrimination in Healthcare Settings Is Associated with Disability in Older Adults: Health and Retirement Study, 2008–2012," *Journal of General Internal Medicine* 30, no. 10 (2015): 1413–20.
35. David A. Ansell and Edwin K. McDonald, "Bias, Black Lives, and Academic Medicine," *New England Journal of Medicine* 372, no. 12 (2015): 1087–89.
36. Institute of Medicine, *America's Uninsured Crisis: Consequences for Health and Health Care* (Washington, DC: National Academies Press, 2009), 60–63.
37. J. Hadley, "Insurance Coverage, Medical Care Use, and Short-Term Health Changes Following an Unintentional Injury or the Onset of a Chronic Condition," *JAMA* 297, no. 10 (2007): 1073–84.
38. Andrew P. Wilper et al., "Health Insurance and Mortality in US Adults," *American Journal of Public Health* 99, no. 12 (2009): 2289–95, DOI: 10.2105/AJPH.2008 .157685, PMCID: PMC2775760, l.
39. Angus Deaton, "What Does the Empirical Evidence Tell Us about the Injustice of Health Inequalities?" in *Inequalities in Health: Concepts, Measures, and Ethics*, ed. Nir Eyal, Samia Hurst, Ole F. Norheim, and Daniel Wikler (New York: Oxford University Press, 2013), 263–81, http://www.princeton.edu/~deaton/downloads /Deaton_What_Does_the_Empirical_Evidence_Tell_Us.pdf.
40. Adil H. Haider et al., "Association between Hospitals Caring for a Disproportionately High Percentage of Minority Trauma Patients and Increased Mortality: A Nationwide Analysis of 434 Hospitals," *Archives of Surgery* 147, no. 1 (2012): 63–70.
41. Ibid.
42. Jonathan Skinner et al., "Mortality after Acute Myocardial Infarction in Hospitals That Disproportionately Treat Black Patients," *Circulation* 112, no. 17 (2005): 2634–41.

43. F. L. Lucas et al., "Race and Surgical Mortality in the United States," *Annals of Surgery* 243, no. 2 (2006): 281.

44. David E. Wang, Yusuke Tsugawa, Jose F. Figueroa, and Ashish K. Jha, "Association between the Centers for Medicare and Medicaid Services Hospital Star Rating and Patient Outcomes," *JAMA Internal Medicine* 176, no. 6 (2016): 848–50.

45. Peter B. Bach et al., "Primary Care Physicians Who Treat Blacks and Whites," *New England Journal of Medicine* 351, no. 6 (2004): 575–84.

46. Illinois Health Facilities and Services Review Board and Illinois Department of Public Health, "Report of Annual Expenditures, 2012," Springfield, IL, November 2013, http://www.illinois.gov/sites/hfsrb/InventoriesData/Revenue/Documents /Capital%20Expenditure%20Report%202012.pdf, accessed June 17, 2016.

47. E. Laflamme, J. Bhatt, A. Hankinson, and K. Bocskay, "Life Expectancy in Chicago, 1990–2010," *Healthy Chicago Reports*, Chicago Department of Public Health, June 2014.

48. Amir A. Ghaferi, John D. Birkmeyer, and Justin B. Dimick, "Variation in Hospital Mortality Associated with Inpatient Surgery," *New England Journal of Medicine* 361, no. 14 (2009): 1368–75.

49. Amir A. Ghaferi, John D. Birkmeyer, and Justin B. Dimick, "Hospital Volume and Failure to Rescue with High-Risk Surgery," *Medical Care* 49, no. 12 (2011): 1076–81.

50. Govind Rangrass, Amir A. Ghaferi, and Justin B. Dimick, "Explaining Racial Disparities in Outcomes after Cardiac Surgery: The Role of Hospital Quality," *JAMA Surgery* 149, no. 3 (2014): 223–27.

51. Csaba P. Kovesdy et al., "Association of Race with Mortality and Cardiovascular Events in a Large Cohort of US Veterans," *Circulation* 132, no. 16 (2015): 1538–48.

52. Smedley et al., "Unequal Treatment."

53. John Z. Ayanian, Bruce E. Landon, Joseph P. Newhouse, and Alan M. Zaslavsky, "Racial and Ethnic Disparities among Enrollees in Medicare Advantage Plans," *New England Journal of Medicine* 371, no. 24 (2014): 2288–97.

54. See www.equityofcare.org/pledge/resources/pledge_to_act.pdf.

Chapter 10

1. Justin Bieber, interview by Vanessa Grigoriadis, *Rolling Stone*, February 16, 2011.

2. Stephanie Marken, "U.S. Uninsured Rate 11.9% in Fourth Quarter of 2015," *Gallup*, January 7, 2016, http://www.gallup.com/poll/188045/uninsured-rate-fourth-quarter -2015.aspx, accessed April 23, 2016.

3. David Blumenthal and Sara R. Collins, "Health Care Coverage under the Affordable Care Act—A Progress Report," *New England Journal of Medicine* 371 (2014): 275–81; Katherine G. Carman, Christine Eibner, and Susan M. Paddock, "Trends in Health Insurance Enrollment, 2013–15," *Health Affairs* 34, no. 6 (2015): 1044–48.

4. "Affordable Care Act Medicaid Expansion," National Conference of State Legislatures, April 15, 2016, http://www.ncsl.org/research/health/affordable-care-act -expansion.aspx.

5. Melissa Majerol, Vann Newkirk, and Rachel Garfield, "The Uninsured: A Primer—

Key Facts about Health Insurance and the Uninsured in the Era of Health Reform," Kaiser Commission on Medicaid and the Uninsured, November 13, 2015.

6. "Summary: H.R. 676, The Expanded & Improved Medicare for All Act," Physicians for a National Health Program, February 12, 2013, http://www.pnhp.org/news/2011 /february/summary-hr-676-the-expanded-improved-medicare-for-all-act.

7. Karen Davis, Cathy Schoen, and Farhan Bandeali, "Medicare: 50 Years of Ensuring Care and Coverage—Report," Commonwealth Fund, April 2015.

8. K. Davis, K. Stremikis, M. M. Doty, and M. A. Zezza, "Medicare Beneficiaries Less Likely to Experience Cost- and Access-Related Problems than Adults with Private Coverage," *Health Affairs Web First*, July 18, 2012.

9. David Himmelstein and Steffie Woolhandler, "The Post-Launch Problem: The Affordable Care Act's Persistently High Administrative Costs," *Health Affairs Blog*, May 27, 2015.

10. "Medicare: 50 Years of Ensuring Coverage and Care," Commonwealth Fund, http:// www.commonwealthfund.org/publications/fund-reports/2015/apr/medicare-50 -years—coverage-and-care, accessed April 26, 2016.

11. Bianca DiJulio et al., "Kaiser Health Tracking Poll: February 2016," Kaiser Family Foundation, February 25, 2016, http://kff.org/global-health-policy/poll-finding /kaiser-health-tracking-poll-february-2016/.

12. Ida Hellander, "A PNHP Response to Recent Criticisms of Single Payer, Medicare for All," Physicians for a National Health Program, February 1, 2016, http://www .pnhp.org/news/2016/february/a-pnhp-response-to-recent-criticisms-of-single -payer-medicare-for-all.

13. Max Fisher, "Here's a Map of the Countries That Provide Universal Health Care (America's Still Not on It)," *Atlantic*, June 28, 2012, http://www.theatlantic.com /international/archive/2012/06/heres-a-map-of-the-countries-that-provide -universal-health-care-americas-still-not-on-it/259153/.

14. Sara Allin, "Does Equity in Healthcare Use Vary across Canadian Provinces?" *Healthcare Policy* 3, no. 4 (2008): 983–99.

15. Sabrina Tavernise, "Disparity in Life Spans of the Rich and the Poor Is Growing," *New York Times*, February 16, 2016, http://www.nytimes.com/2016/02/13/health /disparity-in-life-spans-of-the-rich-and-the-poor-is-growing.html.

16. Kevin M. Gorey et al., "An International Comparison of Cancer Survival: Toronto, Ontario, and Detroit, Michigan, Metropolitan Areas," *American Journal of Public Health* 87, no. 7 (1997): 1156–63.

17. David Squires and Chloe Anderson, "U.S. Health Care from a Global Perspective," Commonwealth Fund, October 8, 2015, http://www.commonwealthfund.org /publications/issue-briefs/2015/oct/us-health-care-from-a-global-perspective.

18. Michael Cooper, "Conservatives Sowed Idea of Health Care Mandate, Only to Spurn It Later," *New York Times*, February 15, 2012. http://www.nytimes.com/2012 /02/15/health/policy/health-care-mandate-was-first-backed-by-conservatives.html.

19. *King et al. v. Burwell, Secretary of Health and Human Services, et al.*, Supreme Court of the United States. argued March 4, 2015, decided June 25, 2015, http:// www.supremecourt.gov/opinions/14pdf/14–114_qol1.pdf; Garrett Epps, "The Af-

fordable Care Act Reaches the U.S. Supreme Court, Again," *Atlantic*, November 7, 2015, http://www.theatlantic.com/politics/archive/2015/11/the-affordable-care-act -reaches-the-supreme-court-again/414762/.

20. Blumenthal and Collins, "Health Care Coverage under the Affordable Care Act."

21. Stacey McMorrow et al., "Uninsurance Disparities Have Narrowed for Black And Hispanic Adults under the Affordable Care Act," *Health Affairs* 34 (2015) 1774–78.

22. Institute of Medicine, Committee on the Consequences of Uninsurance, *Insuring America's Health: Principles and Recommendations* (Washington, DC: National Academies Press).

23. Blumenthal and Collins, "Health Care Coverage under the Affordable Care Act."

24. *Lancet* 374 (December 5, 2009).

25. Amanda Terkel, "Lieberman Pledges to Filibuster House Bill: The Public Option Is 'Unnecessary,'" *ThinkProgress*, November 8, 2009. http://thinkprogress.org /politics/2009/11/08/68348/lieberman-filibuster-public/.

26. Sabrina Tavernise and Robert Gebeloff, "Millions of Poor Are Left Uncovered by Health Law," *New York Times*, October 2, 2013, http://www.nytimes.com/2013 /10/03/health/millions-of-poor-are-left-uncovered-by-health-law.html.

27. Kevin D. Dayaratna, "Studies Show: Medicaid Patients Have Worse Access and Outcomes Than the Privately Insured," *Heritage Foundation Backgrounder*, 2012, 2740.

28. Sandra L. Decker, "In 2011 Nearly One-Third of Physicians Said They Would Not Accept New Medicaid Patients, but Rising Fees May Help," *Health Affairs* 31, no. 8 (2012): 1673–79.

29. Gary Claxton, Larry Levitt, and Michelle Long, "Payments for Cost Sharing Increasing Rapidly over Time," Henry Kaiser Family Foundation, April 12, 2016, http://www.healthsystemtracker.org/insight/payments-for-cost-sharing-increasing -rapidly-over-time/.

30. Matthew Rae et al., "Patient Cost-Sharing in Marketplace Plans, 2016," Henry Kaiser Family Foundation, November 13, 2015, http://kff.org/health-costs/issue-brief /patient-cost-sharing-in-marketplace-plans-2016/2015.

31. Blumenthal and Collins, "Health Care Coverage under the Affordable Care Act."

32. "Obamacare Subsidies," Obamacare Facts, http://obamacarefacts.com/obamacare -subsidies/, accessed April 26, 2016.

33. Christopher Flavelle, "Next Health Care Fight? Out-of-Pocket Costs," *Bloomberg View*, September 22, 2015, http://www.bloombergview.com/articles/2015–09–22 /next-health-care-fight-out-of-pocket-costs.

34. Amal N. Trivedi, Amal N., Husein Moloo, and Vincent Mor, "Increased Ambulatory Care Copayments and Hospitalizations among the Elderly," *New England Journal of Medicine* 362, no. 4 (2010): 320–28.

35. Barack Obama, town hall, Madison, WI, 2009, http://www.politifact.com/obama -like-health-care-keep/, accessed April 25, 2016.

36. Bruce Japsen, "UnitedHealth Group May Leave Obamacare Exchanges by 2017," *Forbes*, November 19, 2015. http://www.forbes.com/sites/brucejapsen/2015/11/19 /unitedhealth-group-dogged-by-obamacare-may-leave-exchanges-by-2017.

37. Robert Pear, "Health Insurance Companies Seek Big Rate Increases for 2016," *New York Times*, July 4, 2015, http://www.nytimes.com/2015/07/04/us/health-insurance -companies-seek-big-rate-increases-for-2016.html.

38. "Winston Churchill Quotes," *BrainyQuote*, http://www.brainyquote.com/quotes /quotes/w/winstonchu135259.html, accessed April 26, 2016.

Chapter 11

1. Ta-Nehisi Coates, "The Case for Reparations," *Atlantic*, June 2014, http://www .theatlantic.com/features/archive/2014/05/the-case-for-reparations/361631.

2. Benedict Carey, "Diagnosis: Battered but Vibrant," *New York Times*, January 7, 2013, http://www.nytimes.com/2013/01/08/science/lessons-in-community-from -chicagos-south-side.html.

3. YoChicago, "All about Chicago's Chatham Neighborhood, Part 3," Youtube.com, July 14 2011, https://www.youtube.com/watch?v=4u_oHacHAf0.

4. Wallace Best, "Chatham," in *The Encyclopedia of Chicago*, ed. James R. Grossman, Ann Durkin Keating, and Janice L. Reiff (Chicago: University of Chicago Press, 2005), http://www.encyclopedia.chicagohistory.org/pages/232.html.

5. Carey, "Diagnosis: Battered but Vibrant."

6. Annie Sweeney, "Chatham Residents Team Up against Violence," *Chicago Tribune*, May 16, 2010.

7. "Selected Socioeconomic Indicators in Chicago 2006–2010," Epidemiology and Public Health Informatics, Chicago Department of Public Health, 2011, https:// data.cityofchicago.org/Health-Human-Services/hardship-index/792q-4jtu.

8. Carey, "Diagnosis: Battered but Vibrant"; LISC Chicago's New Communities Program, 2013, http://www.newcommunities.org/communities/littlevillage.

9. Robert J. Sampson, Stephen W. Raudenbush, and Felton Earls, "Neighborhoods and Violent Crime: A Multilevel Study of Collective Efficacy," *Science* 277 (August 15, 1997): 918–24.

10. Carey, "Diagnosis: Battered but Vibrant."

11. Jennifer Clary, "Chicago Neigborhood Indicators," January 9, 2013 (drawn from Social IMPACT Research Center's Analysis of the U.S. Census Bureau's 2000 Decennial Census and 2007–2011 5-Year American Community Survey).

12. Cynthia Todd, "Chicago Suburb Shows Its True Colors; Area Residents Meet to Study Oak Park, a National Model for Integration," *St. Louis Post-Dispatch*, October 10, 1994.

13. David Murray, "The Gatekeeper," *Chicago Reader*, October 26, 2000.

14. Evan McKenzie and Jay Ruby, "Reconsidering The Oak Park Strategy: The Conundrums of Integration," http://astro.temple.edu/~ruby/opp/3qrpt02/finalversion .pdf, accessed April 23, 2016.

15. Clary, "Chicago Neighborhood Indicators."

16. Coates, "Case for Reparations."

17. McKenzie and Ruby, "Reconsidering the Oak Park Strategy."

18. Murray, "Gatekeeper."

19. Tina Reithmaier and Camille Henderson Zorich, "Oak Park, IL," in *The Encyclopedia of Chicago*.

20. Murray, "Gatekeeper."

21. Ibid.

22. Todd, "Chicago Suburb Shows Its True Colors."

23. "Oak Park (Village), Illinois," in *State and County Quick Facts*, US Department of Commerce, May 29, 2015, http://quickfacts.census.gov/qfd/states/17/1754885.html.

24. Robert J. Sampson, *Great American City: Chicago and the Enduring Neighborhood Effect* (Chicago: University of Chicago Press, 2012).

25. Emily Badger, "How Race Still Influences Where We Choose to Live," *Washington Post*, July 17, 2015, https://www.washingtonpost.com/news/wonk/wp/2015/07/17/how-race-still-influences-where-we-chose-to-live/.

26. Murray, "Gatekeeper"; Badger, "How Race Still Influences Where We Choose to Live"; Bryan Miller, "Bobbie Raymond and Her Housing Center: Would Oak Park Have Made It without Them?" *Chicago Reader*, June 23, 1988.

27. Sampson, *Great American City*.

28. Todd, "Chicago Suburb Shows Its True Colors."

29. Ibid.; Sampson, *Great American City*.

30. "Oak Park (Village), Illinois."

31. Cook County Department of Public Health, Epidemiology Department, "Community Profile: Oak Park in Cook County, Illinois, 2006–2008," in *Community Profiles Suburban Cook County 2006–2008*.

32. Chicago Department of Public Health, "Healthy Chicago Reports: Leading Causes of Death in Chicago 2007–2009," September 2013, https://www.cityofchicago.org/content/dam/city/depts/cdph/statistics_and_reports/LeadingCausesofDeathinChicago2007–2009.pdf.

33. Manisha Modi, "Project on Human Development in Chicago Neighborhoods," Surveys Measuring Wellbeing, Center for Health and Wellbeing at Princeton University, March 22, 2001.

34. Sampson, *Great American City*.

35. Felton J. Earls et al., *Project on Human Development in Chicago Neighborhoods (PHDCN): Neighborhood Activity, Wave 2, 1997–2000* (Ann Arbor, MI: Inter-University Consortium for Political and Social Research, April 17, 2006).

36. Sampson, *Great American City*.

37. Kimberly A Lochner et al., "Social Capital and Neighborhood Mortality Rates in Chicago," *Social Science and Medicine* 56, no. 8 (2003): 1797–805.

38. Sampson, *Great American City*; Emily Laflamme et al., *Life Expectancy in Chicago, 1990–2010*, Chicago Department of Public Health, Healthy Chicago Reports, June 2014.

39. Comilla Sasson et al., "Association of Neighborhood Characteristics with Bystander-Initiated CPR," *New England Journal of Medicine* 367, no. 17 (2012): 1607–15.

40. Sampson, *Great American City*; "Community Area 2000 Census Profiles," City of

Chicago, Planning and Development, 2003, http://www.cityofchicago.org/city/en
/depts/dcd/supp_info/community_area_2000censusprofiles.html.

41. Lochner. "Social Capital and Neighborhood Mortality Rates in Chicago"; Sampson, *Great American City.*

42. Sampson, *Great American City,* 154.

43. Neil Pearce and George Davey Smith, "Is Social Capital the Key to Inequalities in Health?," *American Journal of Public Health* 93, no. 1 (January 2003): 122–29.

44. Alesssandra Del Conte, "A Synthesis of MTO Research on Self-Sufficiency, Safety and Health, and Behavior and Delinquency," *Poverty Research News* 5, no. 1 (2001): 3–6; "Moving to Opportunity for Fair Housing Demonstration Program: Final Impacts Evaluation." US Department of Housing and Urban Development, 2011.

45. Alexander Polikoff, *Waiting for Gautreaux: A Story of Segregation, Housing, and the Black Ghetto* (Evanston, IL: Northwestern University Press, 2007).

46. Alexander Polikoff, interview by the author, July 26, 2014.

47. Ludwig Jens, "Neighborhoods, Obesity, and Diabetes—A Randomized Social Experiment." *New England Journal of Medicine* 365 (2011): 1509–19.

48. Ibid.

49. "Moving to Opportunity for Fair Housing Demonstration Program."

50. Jens, "Neighborhoods, Obesity, and Diabetes."

51. Tama Leventhal, "Moving to Opportunity: An Experimental Study on Neighborhood Effects on Mental Health," *American Journal of Public Health* 93, no. 9 (2003): 1576–82.

52. Ibid.

53. Ibid.; Rebecca Flournoy and Irene Yen, *The Influence of Community Factors on Health: An Annotated Bibliography* (Oakland, CA: PolicyLink and California Endowment, 2004).

54. Jens, "Neighborhoods, Obesity, and Diabetes."

55. Jordan Weissmann, "Poor People Live Longer in Rich, Liberal Cities like San Francisco and New York," *Slate,* April 11, 2016.

56. "Geography, Income Play Roles in Life Expectancy, New Stanford Research Shows," *Stanford News,* April 11, 2016, https://news.stanford.edu/2016/04/11 /geography-income-play-roles-in-life-expectancy-new-stanford-research-shows/.

Chapter 12

1. Rosa Parks quoted in "Rosa Parks Quotes," rosaparksfacts.com.

2. Robert J. Sampson, *Great American City: Chicago and the Enduring Neighborhood Effect* (Chicago: University of Chicago Press, 2012).

3. David Ansell et al., "Report from the Field: Illinois Law Opens Door to Kidney Transplants for Undocumented Immigrants," *Health Affairs* 34 (2015): 5781–87.

4. Kari Lydersen, "Chicago without Coal," *Chicago Reader,* October 14, 2010.

5. Ben Joravsky, "Before the Schools, Mayor Emanuel Closed the Clinics," *Chicago Reader,* March 26, 2013.

6. Claire Bushey, "The Rumble and the Reversal, Part 1," *Crain's Chicago Business,*

April 11, 2016. http://www.chicagobusiness.com/section/trauma-protest; Kristen Schorch, "The Rumble and the Reversal, Part 2," *Crain's Chicago Business*, April 11, 2016. http://www.chicagobusiness.com/section/trauma-protest.

7. Ibid.

8. Sampson, *Great American City*; Lydersen, "Chicago without Coal"; Joravsky, "Before the Schools, Mayor Emanuel Closed the Clinics."

9. Beryl Satter, *Family Properties: Race, Real Estate, and the Exploitation of Black Urban America* (New York: Metropolitan Books, 2009).

10. Atif Mian and Amir Sufi, "Chicago and the Causes of the Great Recession," *House of Debt* blog, May 8, 2014, http://houseofdebt.org/2014/05/08/chicago-and-the -causes-of-the-great-recession.html.

11. Dennis Rodkin, "The Foreclosure Crisis Is Still Hurting Black Homeowners in Chicago," *Chicago Magazine*, September 4, 2013.

12. Derek Hyra and Jacob S. Rugh, "The US Great Recession: Exploring Its Association with Black Neighborhood Rise, Decline and Recovery," *Urban Geography*, January 11, 2016.

13. Michael Powell, "Wealth, Race and the Great Recession," *New York Times*, May 17, 2010, http://economix.blogs.nytimes.com/2010/05/17/wealth-race-and-the-great -recession/.

14. Thomas M. Shapiro, Tatjana Meschede, and Sam Osoro, "The Roots of the Widening Racial Wealth Gap: Explaining the Black-White Economic Divide," Institute on Assets and Social Policy, Research Policy and Brief, Brandeis University, February 2013; Laura Sullivan et al., "The Racial Wealth Gap: Why Policy Matters," Demos and Institute on Assets and Social Policy, 2015.

15. Hyra and Rugh, "US Great Recession."

16. Rakesh Kochhar, Richard Fry, and Paul Taylor, "Wealth Gaps Rise to Record Highs between Whites, Blacks, Hispanics," Pew Research Center, July 26, 2011.

17. Satter, *Family Properties*.

18. Sandhya Somashekhar et al., "Black and Unarmed," *Washington Post*, August 8, 2015, http://www.washingtonpost.com/sf/national/2015/08/08/black-and -unarmed/.

19. Kim Janssen, "Michigan Avenue Black Friday Protests Cost Stores 25–50 Percent Of Sales," *Chicago Tribune*, November 30, 2015, http://www.chicagotribune.com /business/ct-black-friday-mag-mile-fallout-1201-biz-20151130-story.html; Aamer Madhani, "Hundreds Protest as Chicago Releases Video of Cop Shooting Teen 16 Times," *USA Today*, November 25, 2015, http://www.usatoday.com/story/news /2015/11/24/chicago-cop-charged-shooting-black-teen-16-times/76303768/.

20. Somashekhar et al., "Black and Unarmed." Madhani, "Hundreds protest as Chicago releases video of cop shooting teen 16 times."

21. Ibid.

22. "About STOP," STOP Chicago, April 11, 2012.

23. Hal Dardick, John Byrne, and Steve Mills, "Mayor Backs $5.5 Million Reparations Deal for Burge Police Torture Victims," *Chicago Tribune*, April 14, 2015, http://

www.chicagotribune.com/news/ct-burge-reparations-emanuel-met-20150414
-story.html.

24. Andrew Schroedter, "Fatal Shootings by Chicago Police: Tops among Biggest U.S. Cities," *Better Government Association, Public Eye*, July 26, 2015, http://www.better gov.org/news/fatal-shootings-by-chicago-police-tops-among-biggest-us-cities.

25. Adam Lidgett, "Police Misconduct Cases Have Cost Chicago $662 Million since 2004: Report," *International Business Times*, March 19, 2016, http://www.ibtimes .com/police-misconduct-cases-have-cost-chicago-662-million-2004-report -2339649. This was not just a Chicago phenomenon. The city of New York paid $1 billion in police brutality settlements between 1998 and 2008. Mary Calvi, "NYPD Paid Nearly $1 Billion to Settle Lawsuits," CBS New York, October 14, 2010, http:// newyork.cbslocal.com/2010/10/14/nypd-paid-nearly-1-billion-to-settle-lawsuits/.

26. Lidgett. "Police Misconduct Cases Have Cost Chicago $662 Million;" Andy Grimm and Fran Spielman, "Racism, Lack of Accountability Plague Chicago Police Department," *Chicago Sun Times*, April 16, 2016, http://chicago.suntimes.com/news /chicago-police-board-releases-accountability-task-force-report/.

27. Grimm and Spielman, "Racism, Lack of Accountability Plague Chicago Police Department."

28. Ibid.

29. "Proven Results in Reducing Violence," Cure Violence, http://cureviolence.org /results/, accessed April 22, 2016.

30. "Cook County Jail 'a Mental Health Provider,' Says Sheriff Tom Dart, Threatening Lawsuit," *Huffington Post*, February 22, 2012, http://www.huffingtonpost.com /2012/02/21/cook-county-jail-a-mental_n_1291851.html.

31. Joravsky, "Before the Schools, Mayor Emanuel Closed the Clinics.

32. Jeffery Bishku-Aykul, "Why Put Trauma Centers Where No One Gets Shot?," *The Nation*, April 29, 2015, http://www.thenation.com/article/why-put-trauma-centers -where-no-one-gets-shot/.

33. Bushey, "The Rumble and the Reversal, Part 1"; Schorch, "The Rumble and the Reversal, Part 2."

34. Bishku-Aykul, "Why Put Trauma Centers Where No One Gets Shot?"

35. Bushey, "The Rumble and the Reversal, Part 1"; Schorch, "The Rumble and the Reversal, Part 2."

36. Satter, *Family Properties*.

37. Ibid.

38. Bruce Jaspen, "ER doctors Condemn University of Chicago Plan to Divert Patients," *Chicago Tribune*, February 20, 2009, http://articles.chicagotribune .com/2009–02–20/news/0902190858_1_emergency-patients-emergency-room -community-hospital/2.

39. Bushey, "The Rumble and the Reversal, Part 1."

40. Bishku-Aykul, "Why Put Trauma Centers Where No One Gets Shot?"

41. Ibid.

42. Ibid.

43. Bushey, "The Rumble and the Reversal, Part 1."
44. Ibid.
45. Marie Crandall et al., "Trauma Deserts: Distance from a Trauma Center, Transport Times, and Mortality from Gunshot Wounds in Chicago," *American Journal of Public Health* 103, no. 6 (2013):1103–9.
46. Ibid.
47. Bishku-Aykul, "Why Put Trauma Centers Where No One Gets Shot?"
48. Bushey, "The Rumble and the Reversal, Part 1"; Schorch, "The Rumble and the Reversal, Part 2."
49. "About #GetCare," Get Care, https://uchicagogetcare.org/about/, accessed April 2, 2016.
50. Schorch. "The Rumble and the Reversal, Part 2."
51. Bushey, "The Rumble and the Reversal, Part 1"; Schorch, "The Rumble and the Reversal, Part 2."
52. Quoted in Schorch, "The Rumble and the Reversal, Part 2."

Chapter 13

1. Martin Luther King Jr., "Remaining Awake through a Great Revolution," speech, National Cathedral, Washington, DC, March 31, 1968.
2. Paul Farmer, *Pathologies of Power: Health, Human Rights, and the New War on the Poor* (Berkeley: University of California Press, 2003); Paul Farmer, "Medicine and Social Justice," *America: The National Catholic Review*, July 15, 1995.
3. Australian Catholic Social Justice Council, Catholic Social Teaching Series, http://www.socialjustice.catholic.org.au/files/Social-Teaching/Reading_the_Signs_of_the_Times.pdf, June 17, 2016.
4. Farmer, *Pathologies of Power*; Beryl Satter, *Family Properties: Race, Real Estate, and the Exploitation of Black Urban America* (New York: Metropolitan Books, 2009).
5. Hal Dardick, "Chicago Mental Health Clinic Closings Spark Opposing Views," *Chicago Tribune*, August 9, 2014. http://www.chicagotribune.com/news/local/politics/chi-chicago-mental-health-clinic-closings-spark-opposing-views-20140819-story.html.
6. Paul A. Jagorsky, "The Architecture of Segregation: Civil Unrest, the Concentration of Poverty and Public Policy," Century Foundation, August 19, 2015, https://tcf.org/content/report/architecture-of-segregation/http://apps.tcf.org/architecture-of-segregation.
7. Ted Howard and Tyler Norris, "Can Hospitals Heal Communities?" Democracy Collaborative, December 2015, http://democracycollaborative.org/content/can-hospitals-heal-americas-communities-0.
8. Ibid.
9. Matthew Desmond, "Eviction and the Reproduction of Urban Poverty," *American Journal of Sociology* 118 (2012): 88–133.

10. Laura Shin, "The Racial Wealth Gap: Why a Typical White Household Has 16 Times the Wealth of a Black One," *Forbes*, March 26, 2015, http://www.forbes.com /sites/laurashin/2015/03/26/the-racial-wealth-gap-why-a-typical-white-household -has-16-times-the-wealth-of-a-black-one/#74ed185f6c5b.

11. "New Report Exposes Damaging Wealth Gap for Women of Color," Diversity, *Forbes Custom*, http://www.forbescustom.com/DiversityPgs/UnityFirst/3.18.10 /DamagingWealthGap.html.

12. "A Short History of Kentucky and Central Appalachia," *Frontline*, PBS, http://www .pbs.org/wgbh/pages/frontline/countryboys/readings/appalachia.html, accessed April 18, 2016.

13. Dylan Matthews, "Everything You Need to Know about the War on Poverty," *Washington Post*, January 28, 2014, https://www.washingtonpost.com/news/wonk /wp/2014/01/08/everything-you-need-to-know-about-the-war-on-poverty/.

14. Shannon Luibrand, "How a Death in Ferguson Sparked a Movement in America," CBS News, August 7, 2015. http://www.cbsnews.com/news/how-the-black-lives -matter-movement-changed-america-one-year-later/.

15. "What Is Single Payer?" Physicians for a National Health Program, http://www .pnhp.org/facts/what-is-single-payer, accessed April 19, 2016.

16. Ta-Nehisi Coates, "The Case for Reparations." *Atlantic*, June 2014, http://www .theatlantic.com/features/archive/2014/05/the-case-for-reparations/361631.

17. Joel Achenbach and Dan Keating, "A New Divide in American Death," *Washington Post*, April 10, 2016, http://www.washingtonpost.com/sf/national/2016/04/10/a-new -divide-in-american-death/.

18. "The Geneva Hippocratic Oath," *Journal of the National Medical Association* 41, no. 5 (September 1949): 225–26.

19. Andrew Steptoe, Angus Deaton, and Arthur A. Stone, "Subjective wellbeing, health, and ageing," *Lancet* 385, no. 9968 (2015): 640–48.

20. Farmer, *Pathologies of Power*.

21. Rebecca Burns, "Undocumented Immigrants Win Access to Organ Transplant Waitlists, and a Shot at Life," *In These Times*, August 8, 2013, http://inthesetimes .com/article/15428/undocumented_hunger_strikers_win_access_to_lifesaving _healthcare.

22. Lisa Clemans-Cope, Matthew Buettgens, and Hannah Recht, "Racial/Ethnic Differences in Uninsurance Rates under the ACA," Urban Institute, 2014, http:// webarchive.urban.org/UploadedPDF/2000046-Racial-Ethnic-Differences-in -Uninsurance-Rates-under-the-ACA.pdf.

23. Ibid.

24. Howard and Norris, "Can Hospitals Heal Communities?"

25. Ibid.

26. Dardick, "Chicago Mental Health Clinic Closings Spark Opposing Views"; David Ansell et al., "Report from the Field: Illinois Law Opens Door to Kidney Transplants for Undocumented Immigrants," *Health Affairs* 34 (2015): 5781–87; Claire Bushey, "The Rumble and the Reversal, Part 1," *Crain's Chicago Business*, April 11,

2016, http://www.chicagobusiness.com/section/trauma-protest; Kristen Schorch, "The Rumble and the Reversal, Part 2," *Crain's Chicago Business*, April 11, 2016, http://www.chicagobusiness.com/section/trauma-protest; Matthew Blake, "Little Village Residents Cheer Coal Plant Closings," *Progress Illinois*, March 1, 2012. http://www.progressillinois.com/posts/content/2012/02/29/pilsen-little-village -residents-cheer-coal-plant-shut-down.

27. Michelle Alexander, *The New Jim Crow: Mass Incarceration in the Age of Color-blindness* (New York: New Press, 2010).

28. Martin Luther King Jr., "Our God Is Marching In," speech, Montgomery, AL, March 25, 1965, https://kinginstitute.stanford.edu/our-god-marching.

INDEX

A page number in *italics* refers to an illustration or its caption.